Evidence-Based
Laboratory Medicine

Bayer HealthCare
Diagnostics Division

Supported by a generous educational grant to AACC Press from Diagnostics Division, Bayer HealthCare

Evidence-Based Laboratory Medicine

From Principles to Outcomes

Edited by

Christopher P. Price,
MA, PhD, DSc, MCB,
FRSC, FRCPath, FACB

Robert H. Christenson,
PhD, DABCC, FACB

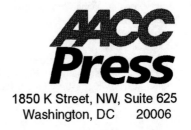

1850 K Street, NW, Suite 625
Washington, DC   20006

©2003 American Association for Clinical Chemistry, Inc. All rights reserved. No part of this publication may be reproduced, stored in a retrieval system, or transmitted in any form by electronic, mechanical, photocopying, or any other means without written permission of the publisher.

2 3 4 5 6 7 8 9 0 G P 06

Printed in the United States of America

Library of Congress Cataloging-in-Publication Data

Evidence-based medicine : from principles to practice / edited by Christopher P. Price,
 Robert H. Christenson.
     p. ; cm.
   Includes index.
   ISBN 1-890883-90-5 (alk. paper)
    1. Evidence-based medicine. I. Price, Christopher P. II. Christenson, Robert H.
    [DNLM: 1. Evidence-Based Medicine. WB 102 E9328 2003]
   RA425.E78 2003
 616—dc21   2003052188

To Ann, Carolyn, and Emma
—CPP

To my mother Deidre and
my best friend John H. (Jack) Driscoll
—RHC

Contents

Preface

Rarely is a career path determined by natural affinity alone. It seems that everyone's professional career is shaped by a series of events, contacts, or experiences that determine which fork in the road to take and determines what will be their focus. This occurrence may involve taking a course that sparked fascination and caused one to "see the light;" another route may be an association with a mentor, family member, or instructor who helped develop a particular interest and served as a role model; the determining event may also take the form of involvement in a project or reading an article or book that changed one's thinking or perspective and developed into a passion. The field of laboratory medicine is no different than any other in this regard, and we suspect that everyone in the profession can recall the event, contact or experience that caused them to cast their lot toward laboratory medicine instead of clinical medicine, basic science, or another field of endeavor.

Once a career path is chosen, the journey begins; for success, the learning experience must be continuous. Beginning in training, there are sentinel events which serve to mold one's career, and all along the way these events shape how we react to problems, our approach to situations and scenarios, and indeed, how we view the role of laboratory medicine in the local and overall healthcare system. One such profound experience occurred for many with exposure to the book *Beyond Normality* by Drs. Galen and Gambino. This book, published as a single edition in 1974, explained very clearly the concept of diagnostic sensitivity, specificity, positive predictive value, negative predictive value, the importance of considering the population at hand, and so on. In part, this book helped a generation of laboratorians think differently about how to interpret the results of laboratory tests. A component of what made this work particularly powerful was the approach; key points were illustrated by very clear examples. An important objective of *Evidence-Based Laboratory Medicine* is to use this same approach to bring relevant concepts into the laboratorian's perspective and into the processes of diagnosis, prognosis, monitoring the effectiveness of intervention, and assessing the effects of intervention.

The origin of evidence-based medicine has its roots in clinical epidemiology. As in all specialties, laboratory medicine involves the interplay between the logic, objectivity, and knowledge base of "science," with the "art" of intuition and feelings that cannot be explained. The "four-letter word" bias is a haze that frequently clouds the reasoning process in patient care, unless these preconceived notions are recognized and cleared to the extent possible. An important intention of *Evidence-Based Laboratory Medicine* is to share techniques and provide a means for compensating for bias, while at the same time merging the science and art aspects of improving patient outcomes.

Part of the attraction of laboratory medicine must be that the field bridges what can be an abyss between bench research and the patient's bedside. This translation process involves a myriad of technical challenges driven primarily by clinical need and includes defining the test's performance in a variety of clinical conditions, evaluating clinical impact, assessing cost-effectiveness, and how clinical decision making is affected by provision of laboratory data. Another compelling attraction of the field of laboratory medicine is the diversity, breadth, and variety of the tasks and activities. This diversity, however, has two cutting edges in that an outcome can be loss of focus on fundamental issues. For example, the technical and financial aspects of day-to-day laboratory testing are clearly critical issues; however, focus on these aspects must not be at the expense of losing the perspective of the patient. A fundamental constant must be the "medicine" in laboratory medicine, which mandates our viewing test interpretation and need from the perspective of the clinical physician. From this perspective, information from the laboratory request will be used in the effort to improve patient outcomes and comprises the Bayesian approach in which pretest probability for a disease or condition is determined, followed by collecting information, i.e., laboratory data, that is proven useful for either increasing or decreasing the likelihood that the pretest notion is ruled in or ruled out. Emphasis on this aspect of the laboratorian's tasks is a major objective of *Evidence-Based Laboratory Medicine*.

There are occasionally events and experiences that serve to refine the thinking process and cause one to "see the light." Our sincere hope is that *Evidence-Based Laboratory Medicine* will serve as such an experience.

Christopher P. Price
Robert H. Christenson

Editors

Christopher P. Price, MA, PhD, DSc, MCB, FRSC, FRCPath, FACB
Vice President, Global Clinical Research
Diagnostics Division, Bayer HealthCare
Newbury, Berkshire
  and Visiting Professor in Clinical Biochemistry
University of Oxford
Oxford
United Kingdom

Robert H. Christenson, PhD, DABCC, FACB
Professor of Pathology
Professor of Medical and Research Technology
Director, Rapid Response Laboratories
University of Maryland School of Medicine
Baltimore, Maryland
United States of America

Contributors

Julian H. Barth, MD, FRCP, FRCPath
Consultant in Chemical Pathology & Metabolic Medicine
Department of Clinical Biochemistry & Immunology
Leeds Teaching Hospitals NHS Trust
Leeds
United Kingdom

Patrick M.M. Bossuyt, PhD
Professor of Clinical Epidemiology
Department of Clinical Epidemiology & Biostatistics
Academic Medical Center
University of Amsterdam
Amsterdam
The Netherlands

James C. Boyd, MD
Associate Professor
Department of Pathology
University of Virginia Health System
Charlottesville, Virginia
United States of America

David E. Bruns, MD
Professor, Department of Pathology
University of Virginia Medical School
Charlottesville, Virginia
   and Editor, *Clinical Chemistry*
American Association for Clinical Chemistry, Inc.
Washington, DC
United States of America

Robert H. Christenson, PhD, DABCC, FACB
Professor of Pathology
Professor of Medical and Research Technology
Director, Rapid Response Laboratories
University of Maryland School of Medicine
Baltimore, Maryland
United States of America

Jonathan J. Deeks, MSc
Senior Research Biostatistician
Screening and Test Evaluation Program
School of Public Health
University of Sydney
New South Wales
Australia

Show-Hong Duh, PhD, DABCC
Assistant Professor of Pathology
University of Maryland School of Medicine
Associate Director, Rapid Response Laboratories
Baltimore, Maryland
United States of America

Matthias Egger, MD, MSc, MFPHM
Professor of Clinical Epidemiology
Department of Social Medicine
University of Bristol
Bristol
United Kingdom

Gordon H. Guyatt, MD, MSc
Professor
Department of Clinical Epidemiology and Biostatistics
    and Department of Medicine
Faculty of Health Sciences
McMaster University
Hamilton, Ontario
Canada

John R. Hess, MD, MPH, FACP, FAAAS
Professor of Pathology and Medicine
Department of Pathology
University of Maryland Medical System
Baltimore, Maryland
United States of America

Andrea Rita Horvath, MD, PhD, EurClinChem, FRCPath
Professor of Laboratory Medicine
Director, Department of Clinical Chemistry
University of Szeged, Faculty of Medicine
Szeged
Hungary

Elaine Kling, MD
Resident Physician
Department of Pathology
University of Maryland Medical System
Baltimore, Maryland
United States of America

Atle Klovning, MD
Specialist in Family Medicine/General Practice
Associate Professor, Section for General Practice
Department of Public Health and Primary Health Care
University of Bergen
    and General Practitioner/Family Physician
Olsvik Health Centre
Bergen
Norway

Deborah A. Marshall, PhD
Assistant Professor
Department of Clinical Epidemiology and Biostatistics
McMaster University
    and Associate Member
Centre for Evaluation of Medicines
St. Joseph's Hospital
Hamilton, Ontario
Canada

Victor M. Montori, MD, MSc
Assistant Professor of Medicine
Division of Endocrinology and Internal Medicine
Mayo Clinic
Rochester, Minnesota
United States of America

Bernie J. O'Brien, PhD
Professor
Department of Clinical Epidemiology and Biostatistics
McMaster University
    and Associate Director
Centre for Evaluation of Medicines
St. Joseph's Hospital
Hamilton, Ontario
Canada

Wytze P. Oosterhuis, MD, PhD
Specialist in Laboratory and Clinical Epidemiology
Department of Clinical Chemistry
St. Elisabeth Hospital
Tilburg
The Netherlands

Daniel Pewsner, MD
Senior Research Fellow in Clinical Epidemiology
Department of Social & Preventive Medicine
University of Berne
Berne
Switzerland

Christopher P. Price, MA, PhD, DSc, MCB, FRSC, FRCPath, FACB
Vice President, Global Clinical Research
Diagnostics Division, Bayer HealthCare
Newbury, Berkshire
   and Visiting Professor in Clinical Biochemistry
University of Oxford
Oxford
United Kingdom

Sverre Sandberg, MD, PhD
Senior Consultant
Laboratory of Clinical Biochemistry
Haukeland University Hospital
   and Professor
NOKLUS
Section for General Practice
Department of Public Health and Primary Health Care
University of Bergen
Bergen
Norway

Andrew St. John, PhD, MAACB
Consultant
ARC Consulting
Highgate
W. Australia

1

Evidence-Based Medicine and the Diagnostic Process

Victor M. Montori and Gordon H. Guyatt

This chapter focuses on the principles of evidence-based medicine with special attention to diagnosis. Diagnostic testing is the process of obtaining information about the patient's health (through history taking, physical examination, imaging, and tissue sample analyses) to discover the underlying cause of the patient's problem. The emphasis will be on laboratory tests, but the principles apply to all forms of diagnostic tests.

THE DIAGNOSTIC TEST

There are two fundamentally different purposes for obtaining a test:

- The first is to detect and establish the magnitude of a physiological derangement.
- The second is to make diagnoses.

The extent to which a test result falls outside the normal range provides information on the severity of the physiological derangement. Clinicians in acute and critical care settings frequently monitor patient physiology using laboratory tests and intervene on abnormal test results to prevent or ameliorate the immediate adverse consequences of these abnormal physiological states. For instance, in the management of a patient with diabetic ketoacidosis in the intensive care unit, clinicians would need to measure pH, electrolytes, and glucose repeatedly to monitor how the patient is responding to therapy and to determine if new derangements (such as abnormal potassium levels or renal failure) emerge. The second use of a test is to make the diagnosis of a certain condition (target disorder), that is, to separate those with the disease of interest (or target-positive patients) from those without the disease of interest (or target-negative patients). For example, in the patient with diabetic ketoacidosis, this diagnosis was established several years ago with two values of fasting glucose greater than 127 mg/dL (7.0 mmol/L).

THE DEFINITION OF NORMAL

The normal range is not very useful in diagnosis because, aside from screening, clinicians do not need test results to distinguish normal people from target-positive patients (Figure 1, Panel A). Rather, clinicians are interested in distinguishing target-positive patients from target-negative patients that present with symptoms and signs that might be attributed to the target disorder. Target-negative patients who, on the basis of their presentation might be confused with target-positive patients, are likely to have test results that differ substantially from normal asymptomatic individuals (and may not differ all that much from results in target-positive patients) (Figure 1, Panel B).

Another definition of normal, the risk factor definition, identifies test results associated with increasing risk of an adverse outcome. In the case of anemia, a prospective observational study of healthy elderly people showed that hemoglobin values below 130 g/L (13.0 g/dL) in men and 120 g/L (12.0 g/dL) in women were associated with double the risk of dying in the next 5 years compared to people without anemia (RR 2.21, 95% CI 1.37–3.57) (1).

Because the relationship between test results and the adverse outcome is usually continuous, it may be difficult to identify a cutoff above or below which prognosis changes. For instance, fasting glycemia is a continuous risk factor for heart disease with values in the normal range associated with an increased risk of coronary events (2).

The risk factor definition does not necessarily imply a benefit in correcting the derangement [traditional blood transfusion practices did not improve, and may increase, mortality in critically ill patients with anemia (3); cardiovascular outcomes do not seem improved when glycemia is lowered to the normal range with intensive therapy (4)]. The therapeutic definition of normal, in contrast, identifies test values for which therapy improves outcomes. For instance, after publication of the 4S trial (5), clinicians considered myocardial infarction survivors with LDL cholesterol concentrations greater than 130 mg/dL (3.37 mmol/L) candidates for statins, a family of cholesterol-lowering drugs. After the CARE trial (6), the LDL concentration above which statins seemed beneficial became 100 mg/dL (2.59 mmol/L). The Heart Protection Study showed no threshold for LDL cholesterol below which patients did not benefit from statins (7). As this example illustrates, the therapeutic definition of normal evolves with the evidence about treatment efficacy.

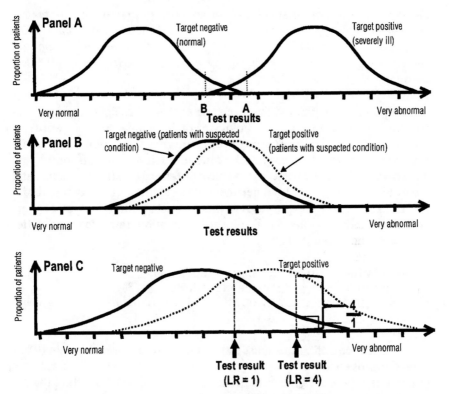

Figure 1 The relationship between patient spectrum and test properties. A: Comparing patients with severe disease with normal people. B: Comparing appropriate spectra of target-positive and target-negative patients. C: The effect of spectrum on estimates of likelihood ratio.

THE DIAGNOSTIC PROCESS

What is the diagnostic definition of normal? This definition refers to changes in the probability of the target disorder associated with different test results. To illustrate, consider the following three patients:

A 65-year-old man of Italian origin and in apparent good health presents with fatigue. He denies overt bleeding, black stools, hematuria, or any bleeding disorder. His hemoglobin is 10.0 g/dL (100 g/L).

A 65-year-old man also presents with fatigue and with a hemoglobin of 10.0 g/dL (100 g/L). In addition, he has a history of active rheumatoid arthritis treated with nonsteroidal anti-inflammatory agents. He has no history of gastrointestinal ulcers, and he uses a proton pump inhibitor to prevent them.

The third patient is of the same age and sex and he too presents with fatigue and a hemoglobin of 10.0 g/dL (100 g/L). He had a colon polyp removed 10 years ago, but he has no history of overt gastrointestinal bleeding. He has not had any other diseases and does not use medications. His father had colon cancer.

Consider the likelihood that each one of these three patients with anemia has iron deficiency as the etiology of their anemia. In other words, in 100 patients like each one of these three men, what proportion would be expected to have iron deficiency as the cause of their anemia? In considering these probabilities, the clinician may have questions about the personal and family history as well as about pertinent physical findings and other laboratory test results. For the purposes of this exercise, assume that the answers provide no additional helpful diagnostic information. Indicate probabilities using the range from 0 to 100%:

1. Man of Italian origin with anemia and fatigue ____ %
2. Man with anemia and rheumatoid arthritis ____ %
3. Man with anemia, history of colon polyp, and family history of colon cancer ____ %

As is evident, clinicians must estimate the pretest probability to determine the probability that the target disorder is present after obtaining the test results. The Bayes theorem describes how the probability that the patient has a target disorder will be revised (upward, no change, or downward) because of the test result.

Clinicians can estimate pretest probabilities using their knowledge of differential diagnosis, their clinical intuition, and clinical experience with patients presenting similarly. Alternatively, they can look to studies in which investigators assemble a group of patients presenting similarly, conduct thorough diagnostic investigations, and determine the proportion of patients with the clinical presentation who proved to have the target disorder.

Studies of diagnostic tests may be constructed to provide this sort of information. One such study assembled a group of 259 aged patients presenting with anemia (8). After a thorough diagnostic investigation, 36% of these patients turned out to have iron-deficiency anemia (indicated by depleted iron stores in the bone marrow); the investigators also listed the proportion of patients with other causes of anemia.

Finally, clinical prediction rules provide another alternative. Clinical prediction rules quantify the probability of having a target disorder (the pretest probability for the next test) using clinical features and available laboratory test results (9). Typically, investigators use the results of a range

Table 1
**Posttest probabilities for iron-deficiency anemia given three
different ferritin test results for each patient**

Patient	Ferritin value, ng/mL (μg/L) Normal: 18–200	Probability of iron-deficiency anemia (0–100%)
65-year-old Italian man with fatigue	10	____
	35	____
	80	____
65-year-old man with fatigue and rheumatoid arthritis	10	____
	35	____
	80	____
65-year-old man with fatigue, history of a colon polyp, and father with colon cancer	10	____
	35	____
	80	____

of information to construct statistical models that yield disease probability estimates.

Returning to the clinical problem, the next step is to choose the best test to determine the cause of anemia in each of these three patients. In the electronic reference UpToDate (10), Schrier reviews the evidence and recommends measuring ferritin to diagnose iron-deficiency anemia. Considering the probability of iron-deficiency anemia indicated previously, now complete the right column of Table 1, reestimating the probability of iron-deficiency anemia in the three men given three possible ferritin test results.

The probabilities in the right column of Table 1 sometimes are called posttest probabilities and represent the probability of the target disorder given the pretest probability and the test result. To estimate posttest probability accurately, knowing how the test result modifies the pretest probability is crucial; clinical research studies of diagnostic tests should provide this information.

USERS' GUIDES TO THE DIAGNOSTIC LITERATURE

In the following sections, we follow the Users' Guides to the Medical Literature (11) to direct the process of incorporating research evidence into practice. There are four questions to ask when using evidence from clinical research:

1. Where is the best evidence?
2. Are the results valid?
3. What are the results?
4. Can the results be applied to patient care?

Where Is the Best Evidence?

To quickly retrieve the best available evidence about diagnostic test performance, one should frame the query in an answerable fashion and then consult an evidence repository. For the first patient the question would be "When compared to bone marrow aspiration for iron stores, does ferritin accurately diagnose iron-deficiency anemia in elderly men presenting with anemia?" This question explicitly describes the patients (elderly men presenting with anemia), the exposure (the ferritin test), the comparison exposure (the bone marrow test, the reference standard for iron-deficiency anemia), and the outcome (diagnosis of iron-deficiency anemia). Note that for the second case, the term "rheumatoid arthritis" further characterizes the patient and could be included in the clinical question.

Use this question to guide the search in Medline (nonfiltered and periodically updated electronic database of abstracts of research studies published in more than 4000 biomedical journals). A search strategy containing the expression "ferritin AND iron-deficiency anemia" and using methodological filters for articles on diagnosis (12) yields 76 citations. Because searching Medline is time consuming and inefficient, clinicians can turn to filtered and preappraised evidence sources. One such source is the ACP Journal Club (13) which collates research reports using methodological criteria and clinical relevance from more than 130 high-impact medical journals, continuously updates its database, and consistently presents data using highly structured abstracts which often contain more detail about the methods than the original manuscript. A focused search using the phrase "iron-deficiency anemia" yields five "hits." Consideration of these "hits" indicates two studies worth reviewing: a study of diagnostic tests for the diagnosis of iron-deficiency anemia (8) and a systematic review of such studies (14).

Are the Results Valid?

The following two questions can be used as a guide in assessing the extent to which the methods used protected the study results from the introduction of bias, that is, to assess the validity of the evidence from diagnostic research:

- Did clinicians face diagnostic uncertainty?
- Was there a blind comparison with an independent reference standard applied to all patients?

Figure 1 illustrates the importance of diagnostic uncertainty. If the investigators assembled a group of patients unequivocally affected by the target disorder (target positive) and a group of normal volunteers (target negative), one will find very little overlap in test results between the two groups (Panel A). Because the appropriate target-positive group will be less severely affected patients, and the appropriate target-negative group those with easily confused conditions, using severely affected and normal volunteers will overestimate the test's diagnostic power.

Lijmer et al. (15) reviewed 184 studies of diagnostic tests to determine which methodological aspects impacted on the estimates of diagnostic performance. Studies with inappropriate disease spectrum (that is, assessing the test in a population with severe disease and in normal volunteers) overestimated diagnostic performance threefold [relative diagnostic odds ratio (RDOR) 3.0, 95% CI 2.0–4.5]. Therefore, studies of a nonclinical population generate only preliminary data as to the usefulness of a specific diagnostic test; if the test cannot discriminate between those severely affected and normal volunteers, it is safe to discard.

A study of iron-deficiency anemia in the elderly (8) enrolled 259 consecutive inpatients and outpatients 65 years or older without prior diagnosis of anemia with hemoglobin less than 12.0 g/dL (120 g/L) in men and 11.0 g/dL (110 g/L) in women and in whom the investigators obtained a blood sample for hematological tests and a bone marrow aspirate to determine iron stores. The investigators excluded patients that were too ill, terminal, with recent overt blood loss, or who had recently received a blood transfusion. This population satisfies the first criterion for a study assessing diagnostic test performance: that the diagnostic test is studied in patients in whom the clinician does not know if they have the target condition, the population of interest to clinicians facing diagnostic uncertainty.

Here a pathologist, unaware of the clinical presentation and hematological test results, evaluated the bone marrow aspirates. Therefore, the study satisfies the second criterion for unbiased diagnostic research studies: that the test under evaluation and the reference standard be performed independently. The bone marrow aspiration, the reference standard, involves judging whether there are or are not iron stores in bone marrow aspirates stained with Prussian blue. Because this judgment is susceptible to prior knowledge of the clinical features and available test results, it seems sensible to keep the pathologist blind to these test results. Lijmer et al. found that studies in which interpretation of the reference standard was not blind to the results of the test overestimated diagnostic performance (RDOR 1.3, 95% 1.0–1.9) (15).

Also, the decision to conduct the bone marrow biopsy was made regardless of the hematological test results. The error of using a different reference standard depending on the test result sometimes is called verification bias and may be responsible for overestimating diagnostic performance twofold (RDOR 2.2, 95% 1.5–3.3) (15).

What Are the Results?

When the study methods are likely to guarantee unbiased estimates of each test's diagnostic performance, then the study results can be reviewed (Table 2).

To summarize the results, one could create a single cutoff to calculate sensitivity and specificity, a traditional measure of diagnostic performance. For instance, one could chose a value of 18 as the cutoff, resulting in a test sensitivity of 55% and specificity of 99%, or one could choose a higher cutoff, say 45, resulting in a test sensitivity of 82% and specificity of 90%. Creating arbitrary dichotomies in continuously distributed test results discards important information: a cutoff of 45 calls "positive" all test results of ferritin from 0 to 45, ignoring differences in the magnitude of change in the probability of iron-deficiency anemia associated with values as low as 10 and as high as 45. Also, a test result of 45 is interpreted as "positive" while 46 (a test result that although numerically different carries almost identical information) is interpreted as "negative." Finally, sensitivity and specificity, without further mathematical manipulation, cannot help in making the transition from pretest probabilities to the posttest probabilities.

Likelihood Ratios

As Table 2 suggests, the results of the ferritin test do not indicate whether iron-deficiency anemia is present. What they do accomplish is to modify the pretest probability of that condition, yielding a new posttest probability. The direction and magnitude of this change from pretest to posttest probability are determined by the test's properties, and the property of most

Table 2
Results from the study of the performance of ferritin in diagnosing iron-deficiency anemia (8). Comparison of intervals of ferritin with bone marrow studies for iron stores and corresponding likelihood ratios

Ferritin, ng/mL (μg/L)	Bone marrow results		Likelihood ratios
	Iron absent	Iron present	
> 100	8	108	0.13
46–100	7	7	0.46
19–45	23	13	3.12
≤ 18	47	2	41.47

value is the likelihood ratio (LR). The LR for a given test result is calculated as follows:

$$LR = \frac{\text{proportion of target - positive patients with a particular test result}}{\text{proportion of target - negative patients with the same test result}}$$

Table 2 shows the LR associated with ferritin test results.

The intuitive use of LR considers the following guide:

- LR of >10 or < 0.1 generate large and often conclusive changes from pre- to posttest probability.
- LR of 5–10 and 0.1–0.2 generate moderate shifts in pre- to posttest probability.
- LR of 2–5 and 0.2–0.5 generate small (but sometimes important) changes in probability.
- LR of 1–2 and 0.5–1 alter probability to a small (and rarely important) degree.

A quick inspection of Table 2 indicates that a ferritin value of ≤18 ng/mL (≤18 µg/L) will be quite useful in ruling *in* the diagnosis of iron-deficiency anemia. A ferritin value of >100 ng/mL (>100 µg/L) will be useful in ruling this diagnosis *out*. Table 2 also shows that the use of the LR for many intervals (using many cutoffs) is an improvement over the forced dichotomy required for the calculation of sensitivity and specificity. The number of cutoffs is primarily determined by the data available; if enough information exists, one could potentially have information to calculate an LR for every possible test result.

Quantitatively, clinicians can use online calculators (16), handheld computers (with software such as MedCalc 4.2 for Palm OS produced by M. Tschopp), a handy nomogram (17), or a manual procedure to calculate the posttest probability of the target disorder using the pretest probability and the LR (18):

$$\text{Posttest probability} = \frac{\text{pretest probability} \times LR}{1 + [\text{pretest probability} \times (LR - 1)]}$$

Summaries of similar diagnostic studies with statistical pooling may provide enough information to generate LRs for very narrow intervals of test results and LRs that apply to a wider range of patients in whom the target disorder is suspected. Now turn to the second study available in the ACP Journal Club, a systematic review of all the available evidence of the performance of hematological tests including ferritin for the diagnosis of iron-deficiency anemia (14).

A systematic review summarizes the literature avoiding bias in the selection of studies, in the ascertainment of study methods and data, and in pooling the results. Methods to achieve these goals include:

- establishing explicit criteria for inclusion and exclusion in data extraction and in methodological quality ascertainment by two or more reviewers working independently with high reproducibility studies;
- conducting an exhaustive search for studies;
- judging the application; and
- using appropriate pooling techniques.

The systematic review examining the properties of diagnostic tests for iron deficiency (14) included studies that enrolled a consecutive series of patients at least half of whom received a bone marrow aspiration for iron stores. The investigators searched Medline and the citations in the bibliography of included studies to identify eligible reports. After scanning more than 1100 studies, they identified 55 eligible reports. The reviewers determined the validity of each study by ascertaining whether patients were consecutive (not selected), that they all received the tests of interest, and that each bone marrow aspirate was read by two or more pathologists working independently of each other and blind to the hematology test results. The investigators measured chance-adjusted agreement among reviewers using the κ statistics, closer to 0 meaning poor agreement and values closer to 1.0 indicating perfect agreement. The reviewers deciding on study eligibility and study methodological quality achieved acceptable agreement in their independent judgments with κ between 0.40 and 0.84. In summary, this systematic review implemented adequate strategies to reduce bias.

The reviewers pooled the studies using summary receiver operator characteristics (ROC) curves (Figure 2A) and LR curves (Figure 2B). The results confirm the superiority of ferritin in discriminating patients with iron-deficiency anemia from patients with other causes of anemia compared to other hematological studies (that is, the area under the ROC curve for ferritin (0.95, 95% CI 0.94–0.96) was statistically greater than that for other tests (range 0.62–0.77) with area under the ROC curve of ≤ 0.5 indicating a useless test).

The LR curves (Figure 2B) model the association of each ferritin test result with its associated LR (therefore narrowing each interval to the individual test result). Investigation of between-study differences suggested that the ferritin test performed differently in patients with different conditions, leading the reviewers to categorize the studies into those that focused on patients with inflammatory conditions (renal failure, infection, rheumatoid arthritis, liver disease, inflammatory bowel disease, and malignancy) and those that had studied patients with a mix of other medical conditions. The LR curves suggest that ferritin is a good test for patients with and without inflammatory

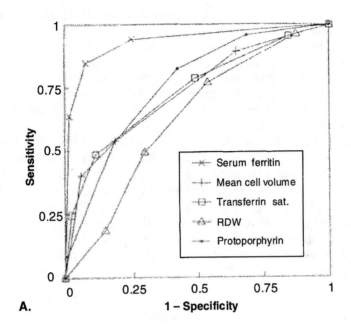

A.

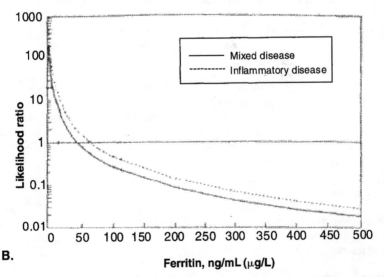

B.

Figure 2 A: The receiver operator characteristics of hematological tests for the diagnosis of iron-deficiency anemia. B: Likelihood ratio lines for ferritin in patients with inflammatory conditions and patients with other medical problems. [Reprinted with permission from Guyatt GH, Oxman AD, Ali M, Willan A, McIlroy W, Patterson C. Laboratory diagnosis of iron-deficiency anemia: an overview. J Gen Intern Med 1992;7:145–53.]

conditions. For a given ferritin test result, however, the LR is higher in patients with inflammatory conditions than in patients without them.

As shown, systematic reviews of diagnostic studies may provide unbiased summaries of the available evidence, precise estimates of diagnostic performance (as illustrated here by the LR curve), summaries that are widely applicable, and information about applicability to specific patients in whom the test performs differently (illustrated here with the generation of LR curves for patients with inflammatory disease).

Returning to the exercise, use the pretest probabilities considered for each of these three cases and the associated LR from the systematic review (noted on Table 3) and calculate the posttest probabilities for iron-deficiency anemia (enter these numbers into the empty cells of Table 3). Then compare these results with the previous estimate of posttest probability (Table 1). Notice the usefulness of presenting the test result in association with the best available estimate of the LR to assist clinicians armed with pretest probabilities in calculating the probability that their patient has the target disorder.

Table 3
Recalculation of posttest probabilities using likelihood ratios from the literature

Case	Pretest probability of iron deficiency anemia (0–100%)	Ferritin value, ng/mL (μg/L)		Posttest probability of iron deficiency anemia (0–100%)
		>100 LR 0.1 46–100 LR 0.4 16–45 LR 4.0 ≤15 LR 54		
65-year-old Italian man with fatigue	____ ____ ____	10 35 80		____ ____ ____
65-year-old man with fatigue and rheumatoid arthritis	____ ____ ____	10 35 80		____ ____ ____
65-year-old man with fatigue, history of a colon polyp, and father with colon cancer	____ ____ ____	10 35 80		____ ____ ____

Can the Results Be Applied to Patient Care?

In deciding whether the results of these studies can be applied to patient care, clinicians may find it useful to think about the following questions:

- Will the reproducibility of the test result and its interpretation be satisfactory in my practice?

If the reproducibility of a test in the study setting is mediocre (because of problems with the test itself) and disagreement between observers is common (because of varying test interpretations), and yet the test still discriminates well between those with and without the target disorder, it is very useful. Under these circumstances, clinicians can be confident the test can be readily applied to their clinical settings.

If reproducibility of a diagnostic test is very high and observer variation is very low, either the test is simple and unambiguous or those interpreting it are highly skilled. If the latter applies, less skilled interpreters in a particular clinical setting may not do as well. Ideally, an article about a diagnostic test will address the reproducibility of the test results using a measure that corrects for agreement by chance (such as the κ statistic). This is especially important when expertise is required in performing or interpreting the test.

- Are the results applicable to patients in my practice?

Test properties may change with a different mix of disease severity or with a different distribution of competing conditions (Figure 1, Panel C). When patients with the target disorder all have severe disease, the LR will move away from a value of 1.0 (sensitivity increases). If patients are all mildly affected, the LR will move toward a value of 1.0 (sensitivity decreases). If patients without the target disorder have competing conditions that mimic the test results seen in patients who do have the target disorder, the LR will move closer to 1.0 and the test will appear less useful (specificity decreases). In a different clinical setting in which fewer of the disease-free patients have these competing conditions, the LR will move away from 1.0 and the test will appear more useful (specificity increases).

If the study does not exactly mimic their clinical practice setting, clinicians should ask whether there are compelling reasons why the results should not be applied to the patients in their practice, either because of the severity of disease in those patients or because the mix of competing conditions is so different that generalization is unwarranted. As already illustrated, the issue of applicability may be resolved if clinicians can find a systematic review that pools the results of a number of studies.

- Will the test results change management strategy?

For any target disorder, there are probabilities below which a clinician would dismiss a diagnosis and order no further tests—the test threshold. Similarly, there are probabilities above which a clinician would consider the diagnosis confirmed and would stop testing and initiate treatment—the treatment threshold. When the probability of the target disorder lies between the test and treatment thresholds, further testing is mandated (Figure 3). Therefore, the management strategy will be determined by the probability of the target disorder (the posttest probability resulting from the effect of the LR on the pretest probability). If most patients have test results with an LR near 1.0, the test will not be very useful (pretest and posttest probabilities will be similar). Thus, the usefulness of a diagnostic test is strongly influenced by the proportion of patients suspected of having the target disorder whose test results have a very high or very low LR. Returning to Table 2, clinicians could expect 77% of their patients with anemia to have ferritin test results that are associated with very high and very low LRs.

Consider the posttest probabilities in Table 4. The probability of iron-deficiency anemia is very high (94%) in the 65-year-old man with fatigue, history of a colon polyp, and father with colon cancer (pretest probability 80%) and a ferritin of 35 ng/mL (µg/L); if another clinician judged the pretest probability in the same patient to be lower (40%), the same test result (35) makes the diagnosis less likely (73%). Therefore, disagreements between clinicians as to what to do after obtaining the same test result in the same patient can stem from differences in their ascertainment of the pretest probabilities. Furthermore, the pretest probability of 80% for the first clinician was not enough to stop testing; for another clinician it may have been high enough to forego the ferritin test and to start testing to determine whether gastrointestinal bleeding explains the iron-deficiency anemia. This

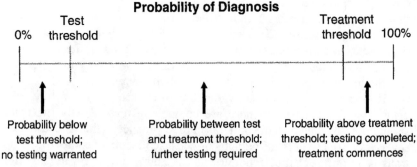

Probability of Diagnosis

| Test | Treatment |
| 0%   threshold | threshold   100% |

Probability below   Probability between test   Probability above treatment
test threshold;   and treatment threshold;   threshold; testing completed;
no testing warranted   further testing required   treatment commences

Figure 3 The test and treatment thresholds. [Reprinted with permission from Jaeschke R, Guyatt GH, Lijmer JG. Diagnostic tests. In: Guyatt GH, Rennie D, eds. Users' guides to the medical literature: a manual of evidence-based clinical practice. Chicago: American Medical Association, 2002:121–40. Copyrighted 2001, American Medical Association.]

Table 4
The interplay of pretest probability, likelihood ratios, and posttest probabilities

Case	Pretest probability, %	Posttest probabilities, %			
		Ferritin 10 LR = 54	Ferritin 35 LR = 4	Ferritin 80 LR = 0.4	Ferritin 120 LR = 0.1
65-year-old Italian man with fatigue	40	97	73	21	6
65-year-old man with fatigue and rheumatoid arthritis	10	86	31	4	1
65-year-old man with fatigue, history of a colon polyp, and father with colon cancer	80	100	94	62	29

additional source of variation in clinical attitude given the same probability of target disorder reflects differences in the test and treatment thresholds (Figure 3).

What determines the test and treatment thresholds? Each threshold implies a trade-off of risks, costs, and benefits. Greater adverse consequences of missing the diagnosis lower the test threshold, while greater invasiveness of further testing raises the test threshold. The test threshold is usually very low for patients presenting to the emergency department with chest pain and suspected of having an acute coronary syndrome because missing a patient with the target disorder can have disastrous sequellae. Similarly, the greater the adverse consequences of a false-positive diagnosis, the higher the treatment threshold; the more invasive the test, the lower the treatment threshold. For instance, the greater the patients' aversion to bone marrow aspiration, the higher the test threshold and the lower the treatment threshold. Because patients live with the outcomes of clinical decisions, their values should play a major role in establishing these trade-offs. Efforts to develop tools to aid in the process of ensuring that patient values drive clinical decision making have focused on treatment decisions with little effort dedicated to the study of patient preferences for diagnostic decision making. Determining patient preferences for decision making in general, and diagnostic decision making in particular, remains a frontier in evidence-based medicine.

• Will the patient be better off as a result of the test?

The ultimate criterion for the usefulness of a diagnostic test is whether the benefits that accrue to patients are greater than the associated risks. How are the benefits and risks of applying a diagnostic test established? The answer lies in thinking of a diagnostic test as a therapeutic maneuver. Definitively establishing whether a test does more good than harm will involve (1) randomizing patients to a diagnostic strategy that includes the test under investigation or to one in which the test is not available and (2) following patients in both groups forward in time to determine the frequency of patient-important outcomes. For instance, patients presenting with apparently operable lung cancer randomized to an investigational strategy that included radiological scanning of head, abdomen, and bones tended to have fewer thoracotomies without cure than patients randomized to an investigational strategy without these tests (19).

When is demonstrating accuracy sufficient to mandate the use of a test, and when does one require a randomized controlled trial? The value of an accurate test will be undisputed when the target disorder is dangerous if left undiagnosed, if the test has acceptable risks, and if effective treatment exists. This is the case of ferritin: the diagnosis of iron-deficiency anemia in the elderly usually reflects a serious cause of blood loss; the ferritin test is simple and has minimal if any risks; and treatment with iron replacement is effective in improving the symptoms of iron deficiency and of anemia. For other tests, confidence in the right management strategy must await the conduct of well-designed and adequately powered randomized trials.

SUMMARY

Some principles of evidence-based medicine have been applied to the diagnostic process. Evidence-based medicine seeks to incorporate the best available evidence from clinical research into clinical decisions. The expression "best available evidence" suggests a hierarchy of evidence determined by the presence of methodological safeguards against bias. This criterion would place studies satisfying all of the validity questions at the top and studies failing to satisfy any question at the bottom of the hierarchy. Because systematic reviews and meta-analyses of such studies include large numbers of patients, they provide more precise estimates of diagnostic power. Because these studies include patients that represent a more complete spectrum of the target disease, their results can be applied to a wider array of such patients suspected of having the target condition. Therefore, systematic reviews of valid research studies stand at the top of a hierarchy of evidence.

Recalling the discussion of test and treatment thresholds, it should be clear that the evidence alone never tells you what to do. In the cases presented, excellent evidence is available for the role of ferritin in diagnosing iron-deficiency anemia. However, the decision whether to investigate further to definitively establish a diagnosis of iron deficiency or to conclude that iron deficiency is present and therefore proceed with investigations such as esophagogastroduodenoscopy and colonoscopy depend both on the posttest probability of iron deficiency and patient values reflected in the test and treatment thresholds.

Finally, the process of incorporation of evidence about diagnostic test accuracy and patient preferences requires clinical judgment and expertise. Without clinical judgment and expertise, a clinician may not understand the true nature of the patient's complaints and inappropriately consider and use tests and their results to guide patient care.

Seeking the evidence, critically appraising it, and judiciously applying it to the specific clinical problem are the fundamental skills for the practice of evidence-based medicine. Health professionals may not have the skills or the time and energy to conduct their own critical appraisal of the original literature (20) and will often benefit from preappraised and filtered resources such as Clinical Evidence (21) and ACP Journal Club (13), or resources that integrate evidence with expert recommendations, such as UptoDate (22). All, however, would benefit from the universal inclusion of likelihood ratios from the best available evidence when laboratories report test results to clinicians and their patients. In the authors' opinion, reporting of likelihood ratios with test results represents that most important step toward the practice of evidence-based laboratory medicine.

REFERENCES

1. Izaks GJ, Westendorp RG, Knook DL. The definition of anemia in older persons. J Am Med Assoc 1999;281:1714–7.
2. Stratton IM, Adler AI, Neil HA, Matthews DH, Manley SE, Cull CA, et al. Association of glycaemia with macrovascular and microvascular complications of type 2 diabetes (UKPDS 35): prospective observational study. Br Med J 2000;321:405–12.
3. Hebert PC, Fergusson DA. Red blood cell transfusions in critically ill patients. J Am Med Assoc 2002;288:1525–6.
4. Intensive blood-glucose control with sulphonylureas or insulin compared with conventional treatment and risk of complications in patients with type 2 diabetes (UKPDS 33). UK Prospective Diabetes Study (UKPDS) Group. Lancet 1998; 352:837–53.
5. Randomised trial of cholesterol lowering in 4444 patients with coronary heart disease: the Scandinavian simvastatin survival study (4S). Lancet 1994;344:1383–9.
6. Sacks FM, Pfeffer MA, Moye LA, Rouleau JL, Rutherford JD, Cole G, et al. The effect of pravastatin on coronary events after myocardial infarction in patients with average cholesterol levels. Cholesterol and recurrent events trial investigators. N Engl J Med 1996;335:1001–9.
7. MRC/BHF Heart protection study of cholesterol lowering with simvastatin in 20,536 high-risk individuals: a randomised placebo-controlled trial. Lancet 2002;360:7–22.
8. Guyatt GH, Patterson C, Ali M, Singer J, Levine M, Turpie I, et al. Diagnosis of iron-deficiency anemia in the elderly. Am J Med 1990;88:205–9.
9. McGinn T, Guyatt GH, Wyer P, Naylor CD, Stiell I. Clinical prediction rules. In: Guyatt GH, Rennie D, eds. Users' guides to the medical literature: a manual for evidence-based clinical practice. Chicago: American Medical Association, 2002:471–83.
10. Schrier SL. Approach to the patient with anemia-I. In: Rose BD, ed. UpToDate. Vol 10. Wellesley, MA: UpToDate; 2002.
11. Jaeschke R, Guyatt GH, Lijmer JG. Diagnostic tests. In: Guyatt GH, Rennie D, eds. Users' guides to the medical literature: a manual of evidence-based clinical practice. Chicago: American Medical Association, 2002:121–40.
12. PubMed clinical queries. National Library of Medicine. Available at: http://www.ncbi.nlm.nih.gov/entrez/query/static/clinical.html (accessed December 2, 2002).
13. ACP Journal Club. American College of Physicians—American Society of Internal Medicine. Available at: http://www.acpjc.org (accessed December 2, 2002).
14. Guyatt GH, Oxman AD, Ali M, Willan A, McIlroy W, Patterson C. Laboratory

diagnosis of iron-deficiency anemia: an overview. J Gen Intern Med 1992;7:145–53.

15. Lijmer JG, Mol BW, Heisterkamp S, Bonsel GJ, Prins MH, van der Meulen JH, et al. Empirical evidence of design-related bias in studies of diagnostic tests. J Am Med Assoc 1999;282:1061–6.
16. Jaeschke R, Guyatt GH, Lijmer JG. Diagnostic tests. JAMA Publishing Group. Available at: http://www.usersguides.org (accessed December 2, 2002).
17. Fagan TJ. Nomogram for Bayes theorem [Letter]. N Engl J Med 1975;293:257.
18. Prasad K. Communicating calculation of posttest probability using likelihood ratio in one step. Br Med J. Available at: http://bmj.com/cgi/eletters/324/7341/824#21308 (accessed December 5, 2002).
19. Guyatt G, Cook DJ, Griffith LE, Miller JD, Winton TL, Casson AG, et al. Surgeons' assessment of symptoms suggesting extrathoracic metastases in patients with lung cancer. Ann Thorac Surg 1999;68:309–15.
20. Guyatt GH, Meade MO, Jaeschke RZ, Cook DJ, Haynes RB. Practitioners of evidence based care. Br Med J 2000;320:954–5.
21. Clinical evidence. BMJ Publishing Group. Available at: http://www.clinicalevidence.com (accessed December 2, 2002).
22. Rose BD, Rush J. UpToDate. Wellesley, MA: UpToDate; 2002.

2

Identifying the Question: The Laboratory's Role in Testing Provisional Assumptions Aimed at Improving Patient Outcomes

Robert H. Christenson, Show-Hong Duh, and Christopher P. Price

This chapter focuses on utilizing laboratory data from individual patients to answer clinical questions that are formulated after assignment of a pretest probability. Clinical questions regarding individuals differ from research questions in that the latter may address basic issues about the pathophysiology of disease processes or may concern more general or global epidemiological issues that require a clinical trial. The focus here will be on clinical care applications; this is an important domain to distinguish from clinical research because, while research question(s) frequently target clinical issues, they do not always address individual patient diagnoses or outcomes.

THE QUESTION IS EVERYTHING (OR IS IT?)

According to the "Standards for Reporting of Diagnostic Accuracy" statement (STARD), research questions are more global and are akin to specific aims, such as estimating diagnostic accuracy or comparing accuracy between tests or across participating groups (1). Research questions are frequently classified according to the following phases (2):

- Phase I: Do patients with the disorder have different test results compared to normals?

- Phase II: Do patients with specified test results have a higher probability of the disorder compared to patients with other results for the test?
- Phase III: Among patients having high pretest probability (that is, the same clinical presentation), does the test distinguish those who have the disorder from those who do not?
- Phase IV: Do patients who have this test measured have better outcomes compared to those who do not?

The results of clinical trials are important to individual patient care; when they are properly designed and conducted to answer clinical research questions, trials provide a most fundamental tool for addressing information needs of individual patients and improving outcomes.

MATCHING THE CLINICAL QUERY WITH THE LABORATORY REPLY

As discussed in chapter 1, physicians and other caregivers obtain diagnostic tests for individual patients to detect physiological derangement, to determine and monitor a derangement's magnitude, to rule in and/or rule out a diagnosis, and to assess prognosis. The basis for obtaining a test is a clinical impression or hypothesis that the diagnostic test will assist the clinician in resolving by adding support, refuting, or providing insight into the ongoing disease process. In this way, the process of requesting a diagnostic test is actually a query, and the test result is a reply. According to Sackett et al. (3), the term 'diagnosis,' or utilization of a diagnostic test, implies not only the decision-making process for elucidating the disease process (i.e., diagnosis), but also for predicting the subsequent course of the disease (i.e., prognosis), for predicting the response to an intervention (i.e., monitoring effectiveness), and for assessing the actual effect of an intervention (3). Table 1 displays examples of questions that drive clinician utilization of diagnostic laboratory tests, frequently in combination with other variables, with the desired outcome that the test result will provide an answer.

As will be discussed later, several questions in Table 1 imply a binary interpretation of the data. The quality of the evidence for the diagnostic test in the context of data from clinical observation and examination (pretest probability) and the clinical question determines the likelihood that the test will assist in the decision-making process and help improve outcome. As in clinical research, examining the diagnostic hypothesis requires questions that are formulated as exactly as possible. Ensuring that the medical laboratory reply is standardized, technically correct, predictable, consistent, and well documented is fundamental, as indicated in Figure 1. However, too frequently laboratory medicine's concern in providing a reply focuses on technical issues and overlooks or loses focus on the primary clinical question that prompted the physician's request. Rather, laboratorians must look at

Table 1
Utilization of clinical laboratory tests for diagnostic decision making

Diagnostic test	Clinical question	Interpretation
Diagnosis		
Intact human chorionic gonadotropin (hCG) in serum	Is this woman of childbearing age, who missed her last menstrual period, pregnant?	Positive or negative
Glucose in plasma	Does the fasting value exceed the threshold for diagnosis of diabetes mellitus in this patient?	≤126 mg/dL or >126 mg/dL (≤7.0 mmol/L or >7.0 mmol/L)
Troponin T or I combined with electrocardio-graphic (ECG) evidence of cardiac ischemia	Does the patient have myocardial infarction?	Above cutoff or below cutoff
Prognosis		
Acetaminophen in blood >4 hr after ingestion	Does this acetaminophen overdose patient have a high probability of hepatic toxicity?	Extrapolate from the Rumack-Matthew diagram (4)
Serum protein electrophoresis	Does this bone marrow transplant patient have evidence of multiple myeloma recurrence?	Inspect pattern for monoclonal protein
Combination of total cholesterol, HDL, age, gender, and smoking habits	What is this patient's 10-year risk for a cardiac event?	Calculate Framingham risk
Monitoring effectiveness of intervention		
Phenytoin in blood	Is the antiepileptic concentration appropriate to avoid seizures?	Therapeutic range: 10–20 µg/mL (10–20 mg/L)
Thyroid-stimulating hormone	Is thyroid hormone replacement therapy appropriate?	Target range: 0.5–1.5 U/L
Combination of whole blood tacrolimus and serum creatinine	Is this renal transplant patient at high risk of acute organ failure due to elevated tacrolimus concentrations?	Tacrolimus >15.0 ng/mL (>15.0 µg/L)
Effect of intervention		
Platelet count	Has splenectomy been salutary in this patient with idiopathic thrombocytopenia purpura?	Platelet count within normal limits
Prostate specific antigen (PSA)	Does this patient have residual tumor after radical prostatectomy?	PSA concentration undetectable
Intraoperative parathyroid hormone (PTH) measurements	Has all hyperplastic parathyroid tissue been re sected during this surgical intervention?	PTH decreases >50% compared to baseline value in intraoperative samples collected 5–10 min after parathyroid resection (5)

23

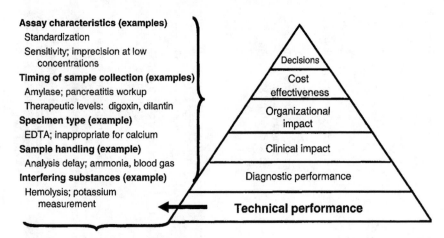

Figure 1 Technical performance is fundamental to the strength of evidence in the process of decision making. (Adapted from Price CP. Evidence-based laboratory medicine: supporting decision-making. Clin Chem 2000;46:1041–51.)

diagnostic problems from the perspective of the treating physician. In this way, diagnostic replies will be clinically focused and integrate into the patient's overall clinical picture, allowing caregivers to make better decisions and take actions that have the best chance of improving the outcome.

FORMING THE CLINICAL QUESTION

Defining the clinical question exactly from the diagnostic hypothesis is essential in the diagnostic process because it provides the means for collecting relevant information. According to the Bayes theorem:

> *If disease was A-fold more probable than no disease before requesting a certain diagnostic test, and if the observed diagnostic test result is B-fold as probable in diseased as in non-diseased subjects, then the disease is (A × B)-fold as probable compared to no disease after the diagnostic test.*

The task of the clinical query is to obtain information that will optimize the B term, in order to have maximal impact on the A term. When the B term is close to unity, that is, equivocal, it will not have large impact, since the product A × B will not be much different from the pretest odds ratio A. However, when the B term is much larger than unity, the product A × B will be much larger than A, and thus the certainty of ruling in a diagnosis will be increased. On the other hand, a B term that is much smaller than unity will make the product A × B substantially smaller than A and increase the certainty of ruling out a diagnosis. The use of D-dimer as a rule out test for pulmonary embolism is the topic of an example in chapter 6 that illustrates this point.

From the caregiver's perspective, producing a patient diagnosis is a process of problem solving that provides a logical explanation for a constellation of signs, symptoms, and other information causative of altered physiological function (6). Cognitive research has shown that diagnostic problems are necessarily approached through a hypothetico-deductive method in which clinicians formulate a narrow range of possibilities, or hypotheses, based on their scientific knowledge, training, experience, and prevailing opinion. The pretest or "working" diagnostic hypothesis sequentially guides the collection of additional information that supports the hypothesis, refutes it, or is unhelpful. According to decision theory, achieving a diagnosis involves updating an opinion with imperfect information (6). Use of the Bayes theorem is essential in that the initial pretest probability from either established disease prevalence or the clinician's opinion is continuously revised and updated as more information is available in what may be conceptualized as a stepwise process.

The panels in Figure 2 show examples (7) of this process in high-risk patients who present to emergency medicine with dyspnea and suspected congestive heart failure (CHF). Data shown in Figure 2A are relevant when the clinician asks the following question on patient presentation: Is B-type natriuretic peptide (BNP) elevated above the established cutoff in this patient with the presenting clinical sign of dyspnea? Using the BNP measurement and a cutoff of greater than 100 pg/mL (>100 ng/L) can either step up the posttest probability of heart failure to over 0.95 or step it down to 0.15. When the clinical presentation and question includes rales in addition to dyspnea (Figure 2B), the pretest probability increases to about 0.70. As shown in Figure 2B, a BNP measurement that is greater than 100 pg/mL (>100 ng/L) results in a posttest probability that exceeds 0.95.

On the other hand, in this same situation, a BNP value of less than 100 pg/mL (<100 ng/L) steps the posttest probability down to about 0.25. Figure 2C shows the effect of adding a third important clinical sign in the context of suspected heart failure, that is, the presence of edema. As shown, the clinical presentation of dyspnea, rales, *and* edema steps the pretest probability to approximately 0.85, a probability level at which some experts suggest laboratory tests add little value. However, as Figure 2C shows, BNP evaluation at the 100-pg/mL (100-ng/L) cutoff adds important decision-making information by either stepping the posttest probability to nearly unity or lowering it to about 0.45.

These examples show that evaluation of clinical signs and symptoms is essential in the physician's stepwise process of determining a pretest probability for whether a patient with shortness of breath as the chief presenting complaint has heart failure. The strength of evidence for BNP is such that the updated posttest probability takes a dramatic step either in sup-

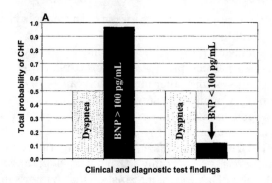

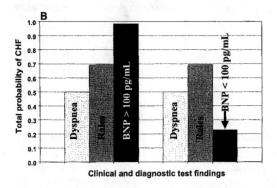

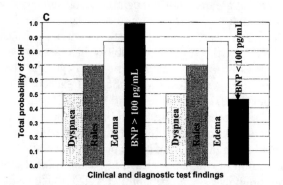

Figure 2 Stepwise process for determining posttest probability using a combination of clinical indictors and B-type natriuretic peptide (BNP) for the assessment of congestive heart failure (CHF) in patients presenting with dyspnea. A: Combination of dyspnea on presentation and BNP result either greater than 100 pg/mL (>100 ng/L) (left bars) or less than 100 pg/mL (<100 ng/L) (right bars). B: Combination of clinical signs of dyspnea, rales, and BNP result of either greater than100 pg/mL (>100 ng/L) (left bars) or less than 100 pg/mL (<100 ng/L) (right bars). C: Combination of clinical signs of dyspnea, rales, edema, and BNP measurement of either greater than 100 pg/mL (>100 ng/L) (left bars) or less than 100 pg/mL (<100 ng/L) (right bars). Data from Maisel et al. (7).

porting or refuting the pretest notion of congestive heart failure as the diagnosis.

Determining pretest probability and cognitive formation of diagnostic hypotheses are based on clinical 'gestalt,' a process that integrates the clinical constellation of biological, physical, and psychological phenomena. Skill in refining a specific hypothesis involves determining what information is useful for developing efficient testing or for questioning competing diagnostic hypotheses, that is, the clinician's process of differential diagnosis. An important caveat to this process involves seeking data that are confirmatory only, acquisition of such redundant information is termed "confirmation bias" (8) or "pseudodiagnosticity" (9). On the other hand, even though confirmation testing may not necessarily increase the posttest probability on a purely mathematical basis, such testing may have value, depending on a physician's level of training, experience, and knowledge because it may improve posttest self-assurance in the result and in any action taken. Another caveat is seeking a test for supporting a hypothesis at the expense of neglecting a competing hypothesis.

Also, it is important to realize that laboratory procedures may not add valuable information to other radiographic, functional, or therapeutic procedures that have already been performed. A particular challenge among clinicians early in training is determining which information is useful in combination with other data, rather than overvaluing any single information set. Optimizing the posttest probability of disease after diagnostic testing, that is, the product of the Bayesian (A × B), is the goal of this process, with critical and thoughtful appraisal of the answer.

ELEMENTS OF THE CLINICAL QUESTION

Diagnostic decision making is frequently a binary process, as illustrated by some of the clinical scenarios listed in Table 1. In fact, the clinical episode for a patient comprises a number of questions with binary diagnostic responses, leading to refined hypotheses and clinical care decisions. Consider the following example involving an end-stage renal failure patient who received a cadaveric kidney transplant. In such patients, caregivers must balance serum creatinine concentrations, a surrogate of renal function [action value: 2.0 mg/dL (177 μmol/L)], and whole blood levels of the immunosuppressive drug tacrolimus [therapeutic range: 8.0–12.0 ng/mL (8.0–12.0 μg/L)]. Tacrolimus is nephrotoxic, so frequent blood measurements are needed to monitor its effectiveness. Serial measurements for both serum creatinine and whole blood tacrolimus are performed daily. The clinician's hypotheses will be modified during the care episode, but in this example the clinical question is to biopsy or not to biopsy. Delayed graft function occurs acutely in approximately 40% of kidney transplant patients and is therefore a primary posttransplant concern for physicians. If evidence of delayed graft function continues for more than 10 days postsurgery, a tissue biopsy is performed and examined by a pathologist as the "reference method" for assessing possible acute graft rejection.

Scenario 1: For 8 days after surgery the patient's serum creatinine levels exceeded 2.2 mg/dL (194 µmol/L); the tacrolimus concentrations ranged from 10 to12 ng/mL (from 10 to 12 µg/L) during this time. On day 9, the patient's creatinine decreased to 1.8 mg/dL (159 µmol/L). The clinical team determined that the graft was functioning and that kidney biopsy was not required.

As already stated, tacrolimus is nephrotoxic and therefore must be monitored carefully. Pathologists can determine on biopsy examination if renal injury is due to overmedication.

Scenario 2: On day 11 postsurgery, the patient's serum creatinine increased from 1.7 to 2.1 mg/dL (from 150 to 186 µmol/L). The tacrolimus level was 18.0 ng/mL (18.0 µg/L)[therapeutic: 8.0–12.0 ng/mL (8.0–12.0 µg/L)]. The clinical team's impression was that the elevated tacrolimus concentration was responsible for the increase in creatinine, and the tacrolimus dosage was decreased. Two days later, on postoperative day 13, the serum creatinine was 2.3 mg/dL (203 µmol/L) and the tacrolimus level was 9.0 ng/mL (9.0 µg/L). A kidney biopsy was performed and was interpreted as consistent with nephrotoxicity due to overmedication with tacrolimus. *The decreased tacrolimus dose was continued at the lower level, and the serum creatinine decreased to 1.9 mg/dL (168 µmol/L) on day 15.*

Scenario 3: On day 19 the patient's serum creatinine was 2.4 mg/dL (212 µmol/L). The patient's tacrolimus level was reported as 4.0 ng/mL (4.0 µg/L), prompting the attending physician to order an increase in the tacrolimus dose. On day 22 the patient's creatinine was 1.8 mg/dL (159 µmol/L), and the tacrolimus level was 11.0 ng/mL (11.0 µg/L). No biopsy is performed.

These scenarios illustrate the interplay between serum creatinine and tacrolimus levels for monitoring the effectiveness of the surgical transplant intervention. Decisions to start therapy, continue therapy, alter therapy, or stop therapy are guided by diagnostic laboratory tests, as well as decisions to utilize an invasive and/or expensive reference method. Often pretest probabilities are reflective of the diagnostic hypothesis, rather than a continuum involving a physiological process. Once the pretest probability of a disease or condition is determined and the hypothesis is tested with laboratory tests, a posttest probability is calculated and the hypothesis can be refined with the development of alternative clinical question(s). Current best evidence for decision making about the diagnosis and care of individual patients demands that the caregiver develop explicit questions, targeting the specific context of the patient. The intention must be that the additional information will play a part in increasing the confidence to use, or not use, a planned intervention or therapy as in this example. There are several key elements and domains to the clinical question, each of which must be carefully identified to avoid spectrum and selection biases (9):

• Population to which the patient belongs
• Prevalence of disease in the specific population (pretest probability)
• Other competing diagnoses
• Confounding clinical conditions
• Pretest Odds Ratio

Matching the individual patient with the population in a body of evidence for the diagnostic test is essential. Therefore, in conducting clinical studies, researchers must take care to match the cohort of patients in whom the question is being asked with the population of individuals for whom the test will be utilized. In other words, interpretation of the diagnostic test must be made within the pretest context (10). For example, meta-analyses including many thousands of patients have been performed on the interpretation and outcome implications of troponin-positive results in acute coronary syndrome patients (11, 12). However interpretation of troponin-positive results in heart failure or renal failure patients in the absence of the acute coronary syndrome is largely unknown. Furthermore, the physiological timing of laboratory testing is a vital component of the clinical question because *when* the specimen for the test is collected plays a critically important role for diagnostic performance (that is, sensitivity, specificity, etc., for interpretation).

Some common examples where timing is important include when to collect specimens for cardiac markers to assess possible myocardial infarction, when amylase or lipase measurements should be performed for assessing pancreatitis, or when specimens for therapeutic drug monitoring should be collected. In the context of acute coronary syndromes, the diagnostic sensitivity of troponin within 3 hours of symptom onset is in the range of 50%, whereas between 9 and 24 hours after the onset of symptoms the diagnostic accuracy approaches 100% in the setting of established cardiac ischemia (13). Thus, the clinical question must be focused on the appropriate contexts of patient population and temporal physiology of the disease process if interpretable results are to be the outcome. Formulating the correct diagnostic hypothesis, determining the correct pretest probability, and obtaining the appropriate laboratory studies to assess the clinical question can all be "trumped" by suboptimal temporal sample collection.

Considering other competing diagnoses is a key element in developing clinical questions. Likelihood ratios for a positive test are often calculated comparing patients having no disease (normal individuals) with those having disease (phase I studies). It may be obvious that a most valuable role for laboratory tests is for evaluating competing diseases and conditions with phase III type questions formulated in the context of patients with the same clinical presentation (high pretest probability), that is, does the test distinguish those who have the disorder from those who do not. Thus, the ability of a diagnostic test to refine the diagnosis or distinguish it from competing diseases and conditions is an important characteristic for effective utilization. As the listing in Table 2 indicates, biological considerations, timing of

Table 2
Key elements for consideration from the laboratory perspective

Timing of samples

Likelihood ratio for the test

Biological characteristics of diagnostic analytes
    Tissue sources
    Tissue/plasma ratio
    Temporal sequence

Preparation of the patient
    Effect of fasting
    Effect of posture
    Effect of exercise
    Effect of age

Technical characteristics of the diagnostic test
    Sample type
    Analyte measurement range
    Clinical measurement range
    Confounding variables (e.g., interference)
    Imprecision (across range of values)
    Accuracy

Diagnostic performance
    Sensitivity
    Specificity
    Positive predictive value
    Negative predictive value

sample collection, specimen type, sample handling, interfering substances, and other technical characteristics influence the results and utility of a diagnostic test. As illustrated in Figure 1, technical performance data such as those listed are the foundation for the decision-making pyramid. Although characteristics such as diagnostic sensitivity and specificity derive from primary studies and meta-analyses, clinical impact and health outcomes, economic considerations and so on all are based on this technical foundation as indicated in Figure 1.

POTENTIAL CLINICAL IMPACT INFLUENCES THE CLINICAL QUERY

Clinicians learn early in training that they must not exclusively focus on the diseases or conditions having the highest pretest probability in individual patients. Even in situations where the pretest probability is relatively low, certain conditions have dire consequences which have a substantial likelihood of bad outcome if left undiagnosed and untreated. A few examples of such conditions include myocardial infarction, stroke, appendicitis, renal failure, and pulmonary embolism. When the pretest probability is low and the consequences of missing the diagnosis are dire, a 'rule-out' test can be used effectively. Disease prevalence is a critical consideration in such situations, as is the interplay between false-negative (diagnostic sensitivity) and false-positive (diagnostic specificity) results.

IDENTIFYING IMPORTANT ELEMENTS IN FORMULATING CLINICAL QUESTIONS

The following exercises are intended to help focus on important clinical questions.

Case 1

A 65-year-old man with a history of hypertension appears in the emergency department with shortness of breath and diaphoresis. The gentleman is 5'10" (178 cm) tall, weighs 245 lb (111 kg), and has smoked two packs of cigarettes per day for 40 years. He had a myocardial infarction (MI) 2 years previously. It is of note that only 3% of the patients arriving in this emergency department are diagnosed as having an MI.

This patient has risk factors including "maleness," a history of MI, older age, obesity, hypertension, and tobacco use. Key clinical elements for this patient include his population and its prevalence and other competing diagnoses. The tentative diagnosis (hypothesis) is that the patient is having an MI. Please fill in the following pretest probability:

Pretest probability of MI _____

A clinician's first question regarding this patient is: Does this patient have electrocardiographic findings indicating an MI? The patient's electrocardiogram (ECG) is performed and interpreted as nondiagnostic. It is important to note that while 90% of patients with a diagnostic ECG are diagnosed as having an MI, only 30–50% of patients who have an MI demonstrate a diagnostic ECG. How does this alter the pretest probability?

MI pretest probability _____

Having the clinical history and ECG in hand, the clinician knows that the definitive test for assessing an MI in the setting of ischemia is troponin and should ask the key question: Does the patient have a positive troponin I result, indicating necrosis and an MI? The cardiac troponin I result is negative for an MI [value = 0.03 ng/mL (0.03 µg/L); cutoff = 0.10 ng/mL (0.10 µg/L)].

Pretest odds ratio _____ × Likelihood ratio _____
                                   =   Posttest odds ratio _____

This case and the queries may seem straightforward, but there are several critical details missing. There are key laboratory elements (Table 2), some of which are omitted from the information provided; one involves timing. Troponin is not an early marker of necrosis (13), and it therefore requires passage of time and appropriate temporal sampling before a negative result is reliable. The laboratory query must be placed in the context of the time course of the event the patient was in. Diagnostic hypotheses involving ruling in of a condition, such as an MI, should ideally be done in a high-prevalence population. In such a case, high specificity (few false positives) is a desirable characteristic for the diagnostic test so that the positive predictive value is maximized.

On the other hand, when hypotheses involve a rule-out test, high sensitivity (few false-negative results) is desirable so that patients having the disease are rarely classified incorrectly as negative. Usually this condition involves a low prevalence population, and diagnostic tests with high sensitivity confer high negative predictive value. In contrast, in a high-prevalence population even tests with high sensitivity do not have high negative predictive value because a substantial proportion of negative results will be falsely so.

Case 2

A 22-year-old woman experiences chest pain and shortness of breath while playing tennis. Nine hours later, at the urging of her husband, she presents to the local emergency department.

How does this patient's risk profile compare to that of the gentleman in Case 1? Again key clinical elements include her population, prevalence of an MI, and other competing diagnoses. The tentative diagnosis (hypothesis) is that the patient is at low risk for an MI, but the condition must be ruled out because the consequences are dire. Please fill in pretest probability:

Pretest probability of MI _____

Does this patient have ECG findings indicating an MI?
The woman's ECG is performed and interpreted as normal. It is important to note that 2% of patients who are diagnosed as having an MI have a normal ECG. How does this alter the pretest probability?

MI pretest probability _____

Having the clinical history and ECG in hand, the clinician knows that the definitive test for assessing an MI in the setting of ischemia is troponin and should ask the key question: Does the patient have a negative troponin I result, ruling out necrosis and an MI?

The cardiac troponin I result is elevated [value = 0.12 ng/mL (0.12 µg/L); cutoff = 0.10 ng/mL (0.10 µg/L)].

Pretest odds ratio_____ × Likelihood ratio _____
$$= \text{Posttest odds ratio} \_\_\_\_\_$$

It may be a bit difficult to calculate the posttest odds ratio; the difficulty lies in making a troponin result that is just above the cutoff intuitively meaningful on a patient with a normal ECG. The clinical algorithm in this case calls for troponin as a rule-out test since the patient is from a low risk population. In this context, a negative troponin test result rules out the patient from having an MI. On the other hand, a positive result is not very helpful since the positive predictive value is low in such a low MI prevalence population. A strategy that would most probably be used in this situation is to repeat the troponin testing later, realizing that after an MI troponin has a characteristic rise and fall.

Case 3

A 55-year-old woman has a history of sweating extensively at night, heart pal-pitations, anxiety, recent 8.8-lb (4-kg) weight loss, and flushing. Five years ago the patient was diagnosed and treated surgically for thyroid carcinoma and has been prescribed Synthroid (synthetic thyroid hormone) since her sur-gery.

During the patient examination and interview, the clinician determined her blood pressure, finding it to be elevated at 150/90.

Please formulate a plausible diagnostic hypothesis for this case and then es-timate the pretest probability. _____

The treating clinician hypothesizes that the patient's symptoms are because the therapeutic level of thyroid hormone replacement is inappropriately high. He decreases the patient's Synthroid dose and formulates the ques-tion: Does this patient have a biochemical finding (TSH) consistent with ap-propriate suppression of the hypothalamic–thyroid feedback system? The clinician was at first a bit puzzled because the third-generation TSH result for this patient was 0.6 U/L (reference interval: 0.5–3.0 U/L). However, he rationalized that this is close to abnormal and thus in agreement with his hy-pothesis. He requests free thyroxine, total thyroxine, total triiodothyronine, and free triiodothyronine measurements, reasoning that there must be some change in the peripheral conversion of thyroxine. Before the result is returned from the laboratory, the patient is admitted to the local emergency department in hypertensive crisis, blood pressure 200/105. How does this modify the initial hypothesis?

Test results and physiology may not have a continuous linear relation-ship. Technically, the clinician made an error in assuming a near abnormally low result of TSH was in line with a hypothesis of hyperthyroidism (overmedication with Synthroid). In true hyperthyroidism, TSH values tend to be significantly lower than the lower limit of normal reference inter-val, and it is well known that TSH values between hyperthyroid and euthyroid are often represented by the euthyroid sick population. This case also illustrates a more fundamental issue. It is human nature to find what is expected (or hoped) to be found, and unfortunately there is no exemption for this trait in the diagnostic process (2).

In this example, the clinician had expected to find results that were con-sistent with inappropriately high Synthroid administration. This expecta-tion could have biased his interpretation of the TSH result and caused him to be further trapped in the initial hypothesis and sought confirmation,

Table 3
Six strategies for minimizing clinical disagreement [adapted from (3)]

1. Match the diagnostic environment to the diagnostic task.
2. Seek corroboration of key findings.
   Repeat key elements and diagnostic studies.
   Corroborate important findings.
   Confirm key clinical findings with appropriate tests.
   Ask "blinded" colleagues to examine the patient.
3. Report evidence as well as inference, making a clear distinction between the two.
4. Use appropriate technical aids.
5. "Blind" the assessments of raw diagnostic test data.
6. Apply the social sciences, as well as the biological sciences, of medicine.

without modifying the initial hypothesis or considering competing hypotheses. In this case, the history of thyroid carcinoma, along with clinical symptoms should have raised the possibility of an hypothesis that included multiple endocrine neoplasia (MEN), a component of which can be pheochromocytoma. Learning from what may be construed as errors in hypothesis generation and clinical queries is important. Perhaps the clinician could have corroborated the hypertension findings with information from the clinical record. Six strategies for minimizing clinical disagreement that may be viewed as helpful in determining clinical queries have been collated by Sackett et al. (3) and are listed in Table 3.

Case 4

A renal transplant patient receiving the standard course of immunosuppressive therapy was afebrile, had a stable white count, and was progressing well clinically. The patient's serial serum creatinine values were between 1.6 and 1.9 mg/dL (between 141 and 168 μmol/L), and the tacrolimus level was between 9.0 and 11.0 ng/mL (between 9.0 and 11.0 μg/L)[therapeutic range: 8.0–12.0 ng/mL (8.0–12.0 μg/L)] for 5 days postsurgery. On day six while the patient was being prepared for hospital discharge, her serum creatinine value was reported as 5.2 mg/dL (460 μmol/L); the tacrolimus concentration in a sample collected 1 hour after the creatinine level was 10.0 ng/mL (10.0 μg/L).

Pretest probability of rejection _____

What is the next action that should be performed?

Although the patient appeared to be clinically stable, it is well known that immunosuppressive therapy can confound the physiological picture of acute rejection. The nephrologist caring for the patient canceled the discharge and performed a renal biopsy, which was sent to surgical pathology. The biopsy was interpreted as showing "no evidence of acute rejection." A repeat serum creatinine value later on the same day was reported as 1.6 mg/dL (141 μmol/L). Later that day the nephrologist was contacted by the laboratory and notified of a sample misidentification involving his patient. The 5.2-mg/dL (460-μmol/L) result belonged to another patient.

This case illustrates that corroboration of key results can be an important query when encountering unexpected findings. Always keep in mind that an unexpected test result can reflect something other than a change in patient condition; it can also be due to inadvertent irregularity in the testing process. Ascertainment of the truthfulness of an unexpected result is advisable, particularly when the subsequent intervention carries serious consequence. Corroboration can take many forms depending on the case (3), but in this case either contacting the laboratory to question and repeat the result or repeating the test on a new sample may have been beneficial.

SUMMARY

Laboratory medicine bridges clinical knowledge and technical know-how to meet a need for objective physiology-based evaluation that is provided in an organized and consistent way. Importantly, laboratory medicine is a key and very common component of the Bayesian equation: pretest probability odds ratio × likelihood ratio (from laboratory test) = posttest probability. Perhaps the strongest indicator of this point is that nearly all patients have diagnostic laboratory studies during the clinical encounter. Although establishing the technical performance characteristics and proper utilization of laboratory diagnostics is a fundamental part of laboratory medicine, there must be better integration and understanding of the process of developing the clinical diagnostic hypothesis, and subsequent queries to test the hypothesis for the optimal use of diagnostic tests and improvement of outcomes. Following formulation of the diagnostic hypothesis, clinical questions are developed that guide subsequent management of the patient, including treatments and interventions, and then the monitoring of these treatments or interventions. Communication with clinical colleagues can help in understanding their thought processes, optimizing the service that can be delivered to the patient, and ultimately improving health outcomes, delivering cost-effective care, and enhancing the culture of evidence-based clinical decision making.

REFERENCES

1. Bossuyt PM, Reitsma JB, Bruns DE, Gatsonis CA, Glasziou PP, Irwig LM, et al. The STARD statement for reporting studies of diagnostic accuracy: explanation and elaboration. Clin Chem 2003;49:7–18.
2. Sackett DL, Haynes RB. The architecture of diagnostic research. In: Knottnerus JA, ed. The evidence base of clinical diagnosis. London: BMJ Books, 2002:19–38.
3. Sackett DL, Haynes RB, Guyatt GH, Tugwell P. Clinical epidemiology; a basic science for clinical medicine. 2nd ed. Toronto:Little, Brown, 1991:1–441.
4. Rumack BH, Matthew H. Acetaminophen poisoning and toxicity. Pediatrics 1975;55:871–6.
5. Sokoll LJ, Drew H, Udelsman R. Intraoperative parathyroid hormone analysis: a study of 200 cases. Clin Chem 2000; 46:1662–8.
6. Elstein AS, Shulman LS, Sprafka SA. Medical problem solving: an analysis of clinical reasoning. Cambridge: Harvard University Press, 1978.
7. Maisel AS, Krishnaswamy P, Nowak RM, McCord J, Hollander JE, Duc P, et al. Rapid measurement of B-type natriuretic peptide in the emergency diagnosis of heart failure. N Engl J Med 2002;347:161–7.
8. Wolf FM, Gruppen LD, Billi JE. Differential diagnosis and the competing-hypotheses heuristic. A practical approach to judgment under uncertainty and Bayesian probability. J Am Med Assoc 1985;253:2858–62.
9. Kern L, Doherty ME. "Pseudodiagnosticity" in an idealized medical problem-solving environment. J Med Educ 1982;57:100
10. Begg CB. Bias in the selection of diagnostic tests. Statistics Med 1987;6:411–23.
11. Ottani F, Galvani M, Nicolini FA, Ferrini D, Pozzati A, Di Pasquale G, et al. Elevated cardiac troponin levels predict the risk of adverse outcome in patients with acute coronary syndromes. Am Heart J 2000;140:917–27.
12. Heidenreich PA, Alloggiamento T, Melsop K, MacDonald KM, Go AS, Hlatky MA, et al. The prognostic value of troponin in patients with non-ST elevation acute coronary syndromes: a meta-analysis. J Am Coll Cardiol 2001;38:478–85.
13. Christenson RH, Azzazy HME. Biochemical markers of the acute coronary syndrome. Clin Chem 1998;44:1855–64.

3

The Relationship between Test and Outcome

Elaine Kling and John R. Hess

I will apply . . . measures for the benefit of the sick according to my ability and judgment; I will keep them from harm and injustice.—Hippocratic Oath

There are timeless elements in the confrontation of the sick individual and the caregiver. The sick tell caregivers what they think the caregiver needs to know while patients still guard their deepest secrets. Caregivers must try to gather evidence, appraise it critically, and apply it judiciously to the specific clinical problems at hand. The need for judgment and the potential for harm are never far away.

Evidence-based laboratory medicine brings new opportunities and demands. Machines spit out numbers, reports, and images in abundance. The relation of these laboratory results to health or disease is complex. Test precision, accuracy, and ranges of normality and the state of clinical knowledge, the nature of statistical inference, and the natural variability of the clinical course all bear on the relationship between test and outcome.

This chapter focuses on the relationship between laboratory tests and clinical outcome with regard to four specific clinical examples. The examples are chosen from common adult diseases, and the laboratory tests are readily available. The emphasis here is on the performance characteristics of the tests and the nature of the clinical information that links the test result values to diagnosis and prognosis.

TEST AND OUTCOME EXAMPLES

Each of the following four clinical examples starts with a scenario. An individual with a few specified characteristics receives a blood test. Within the example, the scenario is followed by:

- a review of the epidemiology of the clinical condition in question,
- the performance characteristics of the blood test, and
- the clinical interpretation and translation of the result.

These three elements, the pretest (prior) probability, test, and posttest (posterior) probability, come from literature-based evidence. However, the relationship between the posttest probability and a clinical outcome is distorted in practice by a psychosocial context, which includes both patient and caregiver. At the end of the example, the scenario is reviewed to look at how the psychosocial context modifies outcome. Large clinical studies of how specific tests perform within the social contexts of medical care and daily life are the most important products of evidenced-based laboratory medicine.

Scenario 1: John Stone, a 42-year-old executive, had his total cholesterol measured as part of a corporate health-screening program. The nurse at corporate headquarters called Mr. Stone 2 days later and told him that the measured value, 250 mg/dL (6.50 mmol/L), was above the action level of the National Cholesterol Education Program.

Heart attack is the most common cause of death in developed countries. It causes more than 40% of all deaths in the United States (1). The underlying pathophysiology of heart attack is almost always arterial damage associated with the deposition of cholesterol in plaques. Atherosclerosis, the accumulation of these cholesterol plaques in arteries and the resulting disruption of arterial integrity, is also responsible for most strokes, almost all aortic aneurysms, and many lower limb amputations. Atherosclerosis is thus responsible for more than half of all deaths in developed countries. It is also responsible for many people living with the effects of ongoing atherosclerotic disease, such as limited exertional capacity from old heart attacks or paralysis from stroke. Preventing atherosclerosis, as a way of improving national health and productivity, is a major health policy goal of most developed nations.

The relationship between the concentration of cholesterol in serum and the occurrence of critical cardiovascular events such as heart attack, sudden death of cardiac cause, and stroke has been examined in a series of large, prospective, population-based cohort studies. The most important of these studies, the Framingham Heart Study, has been going on for more than 40 years. The Framingham Study has identified a number of risk factors for the development of new atherosclerotic disease in previously healthy adults. The most important of these risk factors are smoking, hypertension, cholesterol, diabetes mellitus, and a family history of heart disease. Individuals with four or more risk factors had an incidence of new heart attack or sudden death of more than 40% in 10 years, whereas those with no risk factors had a less than 2% incidence (2). Together, linear combinations of these risk factors account for 50% of all incident heart disease. Differences in the concentration of serum cholesterol account for about 10% of all new heart disease in these risk prediction models, and because of the wide range of heart disease incidence, a decrease in serum cholesterol of 1% is associated with a 2% stepwise decrease in the risk of heart disease (3). Thus, a 33% reduction in the cholesterol concentration from 250 mg/dL (6.50 mmol/L) to 167 mg/dL (4.34 mmol/L) might be expected to reduce by half the occurrence of new cardiovascular events over the next 10 years; from 30 to 15% in an individual with all of the risk factors or from 4 to 2% in an individual with only an elevated cholesterol.

Measuring elevated cholesterol accurately has turned out to be difficult for several reasons. First, cholesterol is a nutrient and an intermediate metabolite. Cholesterol is consumed in food and made in the liver to support the manufacture of cell membranes and the absorption of lipid-soluble nutrients. Its concentration changes in relation to eating, alcohol consumption, activity, and general metabolic state. Not all patients or screened healthy individuals have baseline cholesterol measurements made under the strict conditions used in the Framingham study which included a 14-hour fast, no alcohol intake for 3 days, regular levels of activity, and in their usual state of health.

Second, total serum cholesterol turns out to be the sum of several lipoprotein cholesterol fractions, including "good" high-density lipoprotein (HDL) cholesterol and "bad" low-density lipoprotein (LDL) cholesterol. The concentrations of HDL cholesterol are largely the result of genetics and activity, whereas the concentrations of LDL cholesterol are more closely related to diet and disease.

Third, even the individual cholesterol fractions, such as the LDL cholesterol, are heterogeneous. A given LDL cholesterol concentration may represent a few saturated LDL particles or a larger number of smaller particles with less cholesterol ester in the particle core. This difference has been detected by screening the sera of the Framingham Offspring Study participants with nuclear magnetic resonance measures of lipoprotein particle subclass concentrations that are independent of cholesterol content (4). In that study, larger numbers of LDL particles were associated with greater mortality. However, this association has not been confirmed in other prospective studies, as has the relationship with total cholesterol.

Finally, measurement error also contributes to the variability seen in measures of total cholesterol, and errors of measurement interact with treatment thresholds. Thus, a patient whose actual cholesterol concentration is near a treatment threshold may be given drugs if the measured value is a little high or dietary advice if it is only slightly lower. To get around this effect, some groups recommend multiple measures to improve measurement precision. Reynolds et al. (5) have shown how the inaccuracies inherent in a single measure of serum cholesterol can lead to 30% of patients who need treatment being denied it and 20% of the rest being treated unnecessarily. Repeating the measure three times is advised to increase measurement precision, but that would only be expected to reduce the number of misclassified individuals by half.

Cholesterol testing is widely viewed as important. It is recommended as part of periodic health screening by the U.S. Joint American Preventive Services Task Force, by the Canadian Task Force on the Periodic Health Examination, by the American College of Physicians, and by the British National Health Service. Once a patient is identified as having elevated serum cholesterol, that individual needs to be brought into the context of medical care as a patient. Someone, a physician, physician's assistant, or nurse practitioner, needs to take a history and perform other screening physical measures. The relationship of the patient to that practitioner is an important consideration. The patient will have many questions to be answered. The practitioner will also have questions that require thoughtful and accurate answers as well as a probable need to repeat the testing at a time when the patient has been fasting and alcohol free. Ideal care will depend on many additional factors and may require long-term treatment and followup. All this medical interaction takes time and occurs in a world where an untreated high cholesterol is considered negligent.

Followup: Mr. Stone stopped by the nurse's office a few days later to thank her for the message. He allowed that his older brother and father are fine and that he has never smoked. His blood pressure was measured as normal, He admitted that, with his wife busy taking care of her sick mother, his daughter's soccer schedule, and his own work, he was eating more fast food and getting less exercise than he would like. He is 20 pounds over his ideal body weight. He promised to tell his family physician about the cholesterol, but said that it was not going to happen before the end of soccer season. The nurse offered to call the doctor herself, but Mr. Stone reiterated that he would handle the situation.

Scenario 2. Jane Smith had breast cancer with metastases to local lymph nodes several years ago. She was treated with lumpectomy, breast and axillary irradiation, and adjuvant chemotherapy. She has been well for 2 years. Now she returns with jaundice and a liver mass. A prothrombin time, ordered to assess the risk of bleeding before a planned needle biopsy of the liver mass, was prolonged at 17 sec. The procedure was canceled.

Surgery and other invasive procedures, performed or contemplated, account for the majority of acute care hospitalizations in the United States.

For all of these procedures, the risk of serious bleeding must be considered. The World Health Organization (WHO) has classified bleeding episodes into four grades: 1 = mild, 2 = moderate not requiring transfusion in the first 24 hours, 3 = moderate requiring transfusion in the first 24 hours, and 4 = severe and immediately life threatening even with transfusion support. In the United States, approximately 2 million people a year sustain WHO grade 3 or 4 bleeding in the course of invasive procedures. Many more patients are at risk for serious bleeding as a result of injury, elective or emergency surgery, and diagnostic or therapeutic invasive procedures.

Because of the high frequency and serious nature of bleeding, physicians screen to find patients with increased bleeding risk. To screen for bleeding disorders generally, most physicians ask about unusual bruising or bleeding with injury, dental procedures, surgery, or childbirth. The history questions are a very sensitive screen for severe congenital bleeding disorders, but such disorders are rare. Acquired bleeding disorders that develop in the course of other illness or injury are much more common and require a constant and high degree of suspicion. Therefore, before invasive procedures with a significant risk of bleeding, physicians often obtain a platelet count, prothrombin time (PT), and partial thromboplastin time (PTT) measurements.

The PT and PTT are measures of plasma coagulation. Whole blood is collected into citrate anticoagulant, and the plasma is separated. The plasma is mixed with a clot-initiating agent, either a complete thromboplastin such as rabbit brain for the PT or a partial thromboplastin such as mica chips for the PTT, and calcium. The time to form a clot is measured either mechanically or optically. In the PT test, the specific protein tissue factor and phospholipid from the rabbit brain activate coagulation factor VII and lead to rapid formation of a clot via the extrinsic pathway in approximately 12 seconds. In the PTT test, the mica chips provide a charged surface, which activates factor XII and leads to the formation of a clot by the intrinsic pathway in about 30 seconds. Reduced concentrations of the factors in the pathways leads to prolongation of these clotting times.

The PT and PTT have been very useful for diagnosing and classifying congenital or acquired disorders of plasma coagulation such as hemophilia or vitamin K deficiency, but as general assays for reduced coagulation activity, they are less useful (6). There are several reasons for this. First, the reagents used in the tests are not standardized. Various lots of rabbit brain or mica chips have different clot-initiating activity and reagent stability is not uniform. Thus, the standard error on normal values is large and factor concentrations can be as low as 25–40% of normal before any abnormality is detected. Second, the resulting clot times are not linearly related to factor concentrations. A 50% reduction of a single factor results in a normal clotting time, but a 25% reduction of two factors can prolong the endpoint. Also, coagulation factors activated early in the process have greater effect than those at the end of the cascade. The PT is quite sensitive to factor VII deficiency and thus useful for monitoring warfarin therapy, but the fibrinogen can be as low as 60 mg/dL without measurable abnormality. Third, the test assays only a portion of the clotting process. Physiologic hemostasis is a function of blood vessel activity, platelet number and function, coagulation factor activity, and fibrinolysis. The PT and PTT measure only fibrin formation and only at a standard temperature.

So the question narrows to the relationship between abnormalities of the PT and clinical bleeding with liver biopsy. Patients who need liver biopsies frequently have prolongation of the PT because of their underlying liver disease. They often have multiple other causes of abnormal hemostasis as well. Several studies have looked at the relationship of prolongations of the PT and clinical bleeding in the course of percutaneous liver biopsy.

A study by Ewe (7) reported a consecutive series of 200 patients undergoing biopsy for liver disease, including patients with fatty liver, cirrhosis, and cancer metastatic to the liver. The biopsies were performed using a 1.8-mm Menghini needle under laparoscopic control. A Menghini needle is a solid stainless steel shaft that is missing half of the cylinder for a short distance back from the sharpened end. When the needle is advanced into a soft organ like liver, the empty space in the cylinder fills with tissue. An overriding steel sheath with a sharpened leading edge cuts off the tissue in the cylinder void and holds it in place while the needle is withdrawn. In the biopsy process, the liver is punctured, and along a 2-cm portion of that puncture, it is lacerated. The laparoscope allows the puncture to be visualized, and the length of time that the needle-stick injury site bleeds is recorded.

There was no correlation between the PT obtained before the procedure and the length of time the biopsy site bled. Only two patients among the 200 bled longer than 15 minutes, for 18 and 30 minutes, and neither required additional treatment. This good outcome occurred despite the facts that no patient was excluded because of too great a prolongation of the PT and no patient had their PT prolongation treated prophylactically with plasma. A plot of the observed relationship between the PT and liver bleeding time is shown in Figure 1.

A second study of screening to prevent bleeding during liver biopsy by McVay and Toy (8) reported on 177 patients with a prolonged PT or PTT or a low platelet count and included 76 patients with a PT prolonged up to 1.5 times the midrange of normal (18.5 sec). The definition of procedure-related bleeding in these patients who underwent "blind" percutaneous liver biopsies was a 2-g/dL decrease in hemoglobin or clinical evidence of bleeding. Only eight patients in the larger group bled, and none of those had a prolonged PT.

A third study by Caturelli et al. (9) examined bleeding in 85 patients undergoing fine-needle aspiration biopsy who had low platelet counts (<50,000) or prolonged PT (>18.5 sec). No patient was treated prophylacti-

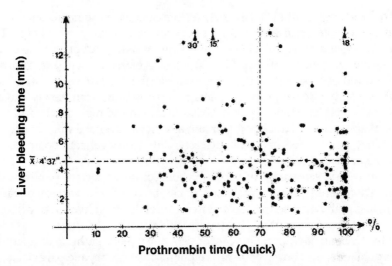

Figure 1 Relationship between the prothrombin time and the laporoscopically observed liver bleeding time after Menghini needle liver biopsy in 200 patients. [Ewe, 1981 (7); used with permission.]

cally with platelets or plasma. No patient had significant bleeding detected by ultrasound.

Followup: After a 2-day delay, Ms. Smith underwent an ultrasound guided fine-needle aspiration biopsy of her liver mass, which revealed metastatic breast cancer. The biopsy was not associated with bleeding.

Scenario 3: Bill Sterling, a 62-year-old black engineering supervisor, sought prostate cancer screening. His internist performed a digital rectal exam that revealed a slightly enlarged prostate. His prostate specific antigen (PSA) was measured at 4.5 µg/L. He was referred to an urologist and underwent six ultrasound-guided transperineal prostatic biopsies (three of the left and three of the right lobe). All of the biopsies were negative for cancer.

Prostate cancer is the most common cancer in men (10). It is the second most common cause of cancer mortality in American men, only exceeded by lung cancer. The incidence of prostate cancer increases markedly with age. It is estimated that prostate cancer develops in one of every six men living to the age of 80. Prostate cancer is present in less than 2% of men between the ages of 40 and 59 years, but it can be found in almost 15% of men between the ages of 60 and 79 years old.

There are marked racial/ethnic differences in the incidence and mortality of prostate cancer (11). Black American men have the highest incidence and age-adjusted mortality rates for prostate cancer in the world (12). The prostate cancer yearly incidence rate is approximately 225 per 100,000 African-American men, 150 per 100,000 white American men, and approximately 100 or less per 100,000 U.S. men of other races or ethnicities (13). The mortality rate for prostate cancer in African-American men is 55.0 per 100,000 versus less than 25 per 100,000 white men and men of other ethnicities. Black men tend to be younger and at a more advanced stage at diagnosis. They have a poorer 5-year disease-related survival rate compared to white Americans (14, 15).

Successful screening for prostate cancer is an important public health goal. Discovered early, prostate cancer can be cured with surgery or radiation, and many men so treated can live entirely normal lives. Early discovery also prevents a particularly painful and distressing form of illness and death. Uncontrolled prostate cancer can cause pain, pathologic fractures, loss of bladder and bowel control, lymphatic obstruction, and paraplegia, all conditions associated with high chronic care costs. Hence, the recognition of the prostate-specific antigen (PSA) test as a highly specific tumor marker was felt to be an important achievement (16).

PSA is a serine protease synthesized in the epithelial cells of the prostate gland. It is usually measured with an enzyme-linked immunosorbant assay and has a within-run reproducibility of 4–7%. Differences between normal individuals in measured concentrations of PSA are greater, both because of differences in the rates of production and removal and in the degree of protein binding. Binding of PSA to plasma anti-proteases, predominantly the α_1-antichymotrypsin, raises total PSA (tPSA) concentration in ways that are not related to its rate of production. Nevertheless, since its introduction in 1987, the tPSA test has become the mainstay of both prostate cancer screening and management (i.e., detecting residual prostate cancer or recurrence after radiation or radical prostatectomy) because of its tissue specificity (17).

The use of PSA for cancer screening when used in combination with either digital rectal examination (DRE) or transrectal ultrasound of the prostate for detecting clinically significant prostate cancer has been validated in large consecutive series and case-control studies of screening (18). The caveat about clinically significant cancer is important because many elderly men die with evidence of low-grade disease that does not seem to have caused them any problems in life. To discover and treat significant disease, the American Cancer Society, the American Urological Association, and the American College of Radiology all recommend that men over the age of 50 have an annual DRE and PSA to screen for prostate cancer. For black men or men with a family history of prostate cancer, they recommended that screening begin at the age of 40.

PSA levels increase with age, mainly because of increases in prostate volume due to benign prostatic hypertrophy (BPH). This led Oesterling et al. (19) to develop age-specific reference ranges for white men from Olmsted County, Minnesota. Others have set similar reference ranges with the study populations still of mainly white men. The upper limits of normal in these reference ranges were set at the 95th percentile of the age cohort value to provide a reasonable trade-off between sensitivity and specificity.

However, among patients with prostate cancer seen in radiation oncology clinics, it has been observed that African-American men have a higher mean serum PSA level even after adjusting for patients' age, tumor stage, and grade (20, 21). In a large study at Walter Reed Army Medical Center, Morgan et al. (22) found that African-Americans had higher serum PSA levels than whites in both prostate cancer and noncancer groups. In this study, areas under the race adjusted receiver operating characteristic (ROC) curves were 0.91 for black men and 0.94 for white men, as compared with ROC scores of 0.70 for Papanicolaou smears for cervical cancer, indicating the value of PSA as a screening tool. Like the Oesterling study, their age-specific reference ranges (22) were set to the 95th percentile, but the reference values (22) are available for white and black Americans (Table 1). Sensitivity was improved among men of the younger age bracket (40–49 years old) and those with an increased risk for prostate cancer. However, in the older age group (70 years old and above) and those with a limited life expectancy, a more specific test is needed. As noted, many elderly patients die with prostate cancer but not of it. Thus, these references should only be used as a guide, with the assumption that associated risk factors and coexisting conditions and the patient's desire to undergo further evaluation are taken into account.

Clinicians should assist patients to decide about screening by discussing with them the options for followup and treatment should a screening test result be positive.

However, screening does become a dilemma because levels can be elevated with cancer as well as with benign conditions, such as benign prostatic hypertrophy (BPH) and prostatitis. Clinical correlation is difficult because the symptoms of prostate cancer are very nonspecific (i.e., urinary hesitancy, poor urine stream, and nocturia) and are also present in benign con-

Table 1
Age-specific reference ranges for the PSA test, based on the 5th percentile of the distribution of PSA level, according to race (22)

Age, years	Whites, μg of PSA/L	Blacks, μg of PSA/L
40–49	0.0–2.5	0.0–2.0
50–59	0.0–3.5	0.0–4.0
60–69	0.0–3.5	0.0–4.5
70–79	0.0–3.5	0.0–5.5

ditions, such as BPH or urethral stricture. The clinician needs to discuss all the options available, including repeating the test after a set time to see if any change has occurred.

Despite the recommendations of the professional organizations, many preventive medicine professionals have argued that the PSA is not a good screening test. A small sample example will demonstrate some of the problems. If four black men at the age of 40 recognize that one will get prostate cancer before the age of 80 and agree to undergo annual screening, the decision has the following consequences. First, they can be expected to undergo 150 tests before one of them, at a mean age of 73, is found to have prostate cancer. The time, medical resources, and financial and environmental costs of driving to the doctor's office 150 times, spending an hour in transit and an hour in the office, and having the testing performed and interpreted are not insubstantial. Second, with the upper limit of normal set at the population 95% point, about seven of those 150 samples collected will have a PSA which falls above the reference ranges. The correct next step for the clinician or patient who gets back a borderline or slightly elevated result, such as a PSA of 3.0 µg/L in a 49-year-old black man, is not known. There is controversy over whether biopsy should be performed immediately or a repeat PSA measured at some interval. Obviously, higher PSA values are of more concern than borderline or marginally high results, but clinicians often feel pressured and pursue biopsy for all patients with even mildly abnormal results. Third, for those with an abnormal PSA, only one in seven will have prostate cancer. A large number of men may undergo an invasive diagnostic procedure with negative results, while risking possible physical consequences (e.g., increased blood loss, infection, or urogenital injury). Fourth, at least some of the prostate cancers discovered will be slow growing and of low metastatic potential. Finding and treating these low grade cancers increases the healthcare burden without necessarily improving the life of the patient. Finally, despite screening, some rapidly growing cancers will occur and spread in the interval between screening visits.

In summary, the PSA is an excellent tumor marker for following cancer patients. However, it has also achieved widespread use as a cancer-screening test without prior validation in prospective randomized trials. In retrospect, it is clear that the area under the ROC curve of the total PSA test is lower than originally reported, perhaps as low as 0.6 in the range of 2–5 µg/L, where PSA raises difficult decisions in screening the aging male population. A better test, based on the calculation of free-PSA derived from the simultaneous measurement of total and bound PSA appears capable of increasing the area under the ROC curve to 0.74 (23). Even with the improved performance, the PSA will still be a test that is expensive and difficult to live with.

Followup: One year later, Mr. Sterling's PSA was 4.7 µg/L. His wife is worried that if he does not get another set of prostate biopsies, he is placing himself at grave risk.

Scenario 4: Brenda Jones, a 66-year-old retired teacher with diabetes developed squeezing chest pain while gardening. She walked to the home of a neighbor who called 911. At the hospital, she was told that she is having a heart attack based on her symptoms, electrocardiographic findings, and an elevated troponin. She was placed in a coronary care unit and immediately scheduled for urgent cardiac catheterization with angioplasty and placement of a stent(s), if indicated.

A heart attack, or acute myocardial infarction, occurs when there is a rapid development of myocardial ischemia caused by rupture of an unstable coronary plaque, thrombus formation, and an imbalance between the oxygen supply and demand in the myocardium. Acute myocardial infarction is part of the "acute coronary syndromes," a continuum of disease that includes unstable angina. The common physiological feature of the acute coronary syndromes is rupture of atheromatous plaques, frequently in the epicardial blood vessels. Thrombus formation in the coronary vessel results in partial or complete occlusion and, in the case of myocardial infarction, cardiac cell death. Total occlusion of a vessel for more than about 30 minutes results in irreversible myocardial necrosis, but urgent reperfusion within 6 hours (and in fact up to 12 hours) can salvage myocardium and reduce morbidity and mortality.

As noted earlier, myocardial infarction is the leading cause of morbidity and mortality in the United States, and approximately 500,000–700,000 deaths are caused by ischemic heart disease in the United States each year. Almost a third of patients with new-onset ischemic heart disease either present with arrhythmia associated sudden death or develop ventricular fibrillation within the first 24 hours. Many such deaths can be prevented by treating or preventing fibrillation. There is a high priority on rapidly diagnosing and treating acute heart attacks.

The World Health Organization's classic definition of acute myocardial infarction requires that at least two of the following three criteria are met: a history of typical symptoms of ischemic chest pain; evolutionary electrocardiogram tracings involving the development of Q waves; and an increase in the cardiac-"selective" creatine kinase-MB (CK-MB) isoenzyme greater than twice the upper reference limit (24). Chest pain is often nonspecific, in that it can occur with cardiac and noncardiac diseases (e.g., pulmonary embolism and gastroesophageal reflux disease). The electrocardiogram is diagnostically specific but quite insensitive, showing diagnostic changes in less than 50% of acute myocardial infarction patients. Therefore, depending solely on evolution of typical electrocardiographic tracings can be detrimental to the patient. With the suspicion of acute myocardial infarction, clinicians often rely on measuring cardiac markers, but the CK-MB has broad normal ranges and is insensitive to relatively small or early heart attacks. The development of serum cardiac troponin T and I assays have allowed the sensitive and specific detection of small amounts of myocardial necrosis. This in turn has prompted a new updated definition of acute myocardial infarction.

The troponin complex is comprised of three proteins designated troponin (Tn) I, TnT, and TnC; this complex is essential for contraction of both skeletal and myocardial striated muscle and is found in high concentration in these tissues (25). Cardiac-specific isoforms of TnT and TnI were discovered and have been isolated; immunoassays for cardiac TnT and cardiac TnI have been developed and these assays have demonstrated excellent performance for clinical assessment of myocardial cell injury (26). On the other hand, TnC exists in the same isoform in both skeletal and myocardial tissue, so measurement of this protein is not clinically helpful.

Cardiac TnT or TnI are present in very low concentrations in blood from normal individuals; these markers show substantial release after myocardial cell death and are therefore both diagnostically sensitive and tissue specific. Following the onset of myocardial injury, cardiac TnT or TnI rise to abnormal concentrations in approximately 3–6 hours following myocardial infarction, with 100% sensitivity being achieved by 9–12 hours. In contrast, CK-MB characteristically reaches a maximum sensitivity of about 90% with serial sampling after about 6–9 hours. Peak values for both cardiac TnT or TnI generally occur after 18–24 hours, and values gradually decline to normal over the next 7–14 days.

It is widely acknowledged that troponin has emerged as an almost perfect surrogate measure of myocardial necrosis. Early studies showed that a cardiac TnI value of less than 0.4 ng/mL is associated with 42-day mortality of less than 1%, but this risk increases progressively to a mortality of 7.5% at a value of 9.0 ng/mL or higher (27). Subsequent studies have shown that even subtle increases in cardiac TnT or TnI in the setting of myocardial ischemia indicate increased risk. This knowledge was, in part, responsible for the redefinition of myocardial infarction by a joint committee of the European Society for Cardiology (ESC) and the American College of Cardiology (ACC) (28). According to this joint effort, the upper reference limit of normal is represented by the troponin concentration at the 99th percentile of a reference control population (28). Many health centers now have replaced CK-MB with troponin as the diagnostic test of choice for myocardial infarction because of its accuracy and relatively straightforward interpretation. The ESC/ACC criteria for myocardial infarction require a single positive troponin within the first 24 hours after symptom onset or a typical rise and fall of the CK-MB with at least one of the following: ischemic symptoms, development of pathological Q waves on the electrocardiogram, electrocardiographic changes indicative of ischemia, or coronary intervention. This (re)definition is able to identify those patients who need urgent care and treatment, as well as aggressive secondary prevention. Identifying these cardiac patients can reduce their morbidity and improve the quality of life.

It should be noted that the psychosocial context of troponin testing benefits the test in clinical practice. The urgency of chest pain, ambulance transport, emergency department protocols implemented by eager young physicians and nurses, full physical exams, electrocardiographic monitoring, and "stat" blood testing gets patients' attention. Few patients wander away too bored or run away too scared or busy to wait for the laboratory answer and subsequent clinical interaction. Also, few emergency department physicians ignore the implications of an elevated cardiac troponin in a patient with chest pain. As a result, the vast majority of patients who arrive at emergency departments with chest pain get "plugged in" to cardiac protocols which are, to a considerable extent, evidence based and known to reduce mortality.

Followup: Ms. Jones underwent cardiac catheterization and was found to have single-vessel coronary artery disease. She underwent percutaneous coronary intervention (angioplasty) and placement of stents without complication.

SUMMARY

Diagnostic laboratory tests represent a major advance of modern medicine. Physicians use them to predict future disease in utero, determine the cause of death postmortem, and for a variety of clinical and public health purposes between. Patients, in turn, see the delivery of their specimens to the laboratory as a personal connection to the large societal investment in modern science. They often believe that their taxes and insurance payments entitle them to tests, as well as to the good health that tests are supposed to bring.

There are several major problems with this view. First, there are many variables that contribute to health and happiness that cannot be measured in the laboratory. Thus, one patient with severe congestive heart failure may view it as a reasonable end to a long and useful life, whereas another may be deeply resentful and angry. Second, even analytes that can be measured well in the laboratory may have little effect on health in many circumstances. The house officer's boast that, "no one dies with abnormal electrolytes on the University Medicine service," probably represents a considerable waste of resources. Third, even lab tests that are clearly related to disease causation and measured at appropriate times may be related to outcome in complex ways. It is in these complex situations that the relation between laboratory tests and clinical outcome needs to be measured with well-designed clinical trials. The Standards for Reporting of Diagnostic Accuracy (STARD) initiative funded by the Dutch Health Care Insurance Board, the International Federation of Clinical Chemistry, the British Medical Research Council's Health Services Research Collaboration, and the Academic Medical Center in Amsterdam is an excellent effort to improve the quality of information available from intervention trials (29).

This chapter examined four examples of common laboratory tests. Total cholesterol is clearly related to the incidence of heart attack and stroke but the relationship is modified by many other factors. Outcome is largely determined by the ability of the physician and patient to use the information provided by the laboratory test to achieve changes in life-style or sustain therapy over decades of treatment. The PT test was designed to help explore the plasma coagulation system. It is now routinely used in clinical medicine to detect coagulopathy prior to minor invasive procedures, but it has little power to do so. The serum PSA concentration is clearly related to prostate size, prostate disease, and prostate tumor mass. Despite the frequency of prostate cancer, using the PSA as a screening test is an expensive strategy that creates a variety of difficult situations. Cardiac TnT or TnI represents an excellent surrogate measure for myocardial necrosis and has become the diagnostic sine qua non for myocardial infarction. Troponin measurement has rapidly spread as the standard of care in the diagnosis of chest pain. The four examples given here are but a snapshot in time of how healthcare providers, patients, and their families use and misuse the information provided by diagnostic tests.

The psychosocial context of testing is also important. The advantages of good information readily available at the critical moment of clinical interaction can be seen in the rapidly evolving use of point-of-care testing in hospitals and clinics. As noted, chest pain patients are not released from the emergency department until their troponin level, along with clinical indicators and electrocardiogram, indicate they are not high-risk patients. On the other hand, there is no evidence that anything should be done to treat a mildly abnormal PT before common invasive procedures. Evidence supports one activity and not the other.

The edifice of evidence-based laboratory medicine is created one good clinical study at a time. Meanwhile, the tests performed and the diseases encountered change. Heart disease has become less common, improvements in treatment have altered the natural history of cancers, increases in longevity make diseases of the aged more important, and rapid diagnostics bring immediate care to affected groups. All of these situations will require new studies in the future and many more clinical scenarios need study now. The collection of high-quality clinical evidence about the relation of tests and clinical outcome will need to continue into the foreseeable future. It will affect the value the patient receives for healthcare investments and the success practitioners feel.

REFERENCES

1. Grundy SM, Balady GJ, Criqui MH, Fletcher G, Greenland P, Hiratzka LF, et al. Primary prevention of coronary heart disease: guidance from Framingham. A statement for healthcare professionals from the AHA Task Force on Risk Reduction. Circulation 1998;97:1876–87.
2. Grover SA, Dorais M, Paradis G, Fodor JG, Frohlich JJ, McPherson R, et al. Lipid screening to prevent coronary artery disease: a quantitative evaluation of evolving guidelines. Can Med Assoc J 2000;163:1263–9
3. Keil U. Coronary heart disease: the role of lipids, hypertension and smoking. Basic Res Cardiol 2000;95 Suppl1:I52–8.
4. Otvos JD, Jeyarajah EJ, Cromwell WC. Measurement issues related to lipoprotein heterogeneity. Am J Cardiol 2002;90(8A):22i–29i.
5. Reynolds TM, Twomey P, Wierzbicki AS. Accuracy of cardiovascular risk estimation for primary prevention in patients without diabetes. J Cardiovasc Risk 2002;9:183–90.
6. Dzik S. The use of blood components prior to invasive bedside procedures: a critical appraisal. In: Mintz PD, ed. Transfusion therapy: clinical principles and practice. Bethesda, MD: AABB Press; 1999.
7. Ewe K. Bleeding after liver biopsy does not correlate with indices of peripheral coagulation. Dig Dis Sci 1981;26:388–93.
8. McVay PA, Toy PTCY. Lack of increased bleeding after liver biopsy in patients with mild hemostatic abnormalities. Am J Clin Pathol 1990;94:747–53.
9. Caturelli E. Squillante MM, Andriulli A, Siena DA, Cellerino C, De Luca F, et al. Fine-needle liver biopsy in patients with severely impaired coagulation. Liver 1993;13:270–3.
10. Parker SL, Tong T, Bolden S, Wingo PA. Cancer statistics, 1996, CA Cancer J Clin 1996;46:5–27.
11. Boring CC, Squires TS, Health CW Jr. Cancer statistics for African Americans. CA Cancer J Clin 1992;42:7–17.
12. Mebane C, Gibbs T, Horm J. Current status of prostate cancer in North American black males. J Natl Med Assoc 1990;82:782–8.
13. Morton RA Jr. Racial differences in adenocarcinoma of the prostate in North American men. Urology 1994;44:637–45.
14. Austin JP, Aziz H, Potters L, Thelmo W, Chen P, Choi K, et al. Diminished survival of young blacks with adenocarcinoma of the prostate. Am J Clin Oncol 1990;13:465–9.
15. Pienta KJ, Demers R, Hoff M, Kau TY, Montie JE, Severson RK. Effect of age and race on the survival of men with prostate cancer in the Metropolitan Detroit tricounty area , 1973 to 1987. Urology 1995;45:93–102.

16. Stamey TA, Yang H, Hay AR. PSA as a serum marker for prostate adenocarcinoma. N Engl J Med 1987;317:909–16.
17. Catalona WJ, Smith DS, Ratliff TL, Basler JW. Detection of organ-confined prostate cancer is increased through prostate-specific antigen-based screening. J Am Med Assoc 1993;270:948–54.
18. Catalona WJ, Smith DS, Ratliff TL, Dodds KM, Coplen DE, Yuan JJ, et al. The measurement of prostate-specific antigen in serum as a screening test for prostate cancer. N Engl J Med 1991;324:1156–61.
19. Oesterling JE, Jacobsen SJ, Chute CG, Guess HA, Girman CJ, Panser LA, et al. Serum prostate-specific antigen in a community-based population of healthy men. Establishment of age-specific reference ranges. J Am Med Assoc 1993;270:860–4.
20. Vijayakumar S, Winter K, Sause W, Gallagher MJ, Michaelski J, Roach M, et al. Prostate specific antigen levels are higher in African-American than white patients in a multicenter registration study; results of RTOG 94-12. Int J Radiat Oncol Biol Phys 1998;40:17–25.
21. Teshima T, Hanlon AM, Hanks GE. Pretreatment prostate-specific antigen values in patients with prostate cancer; 1989 patterns of care study process survey. Int J Radiat Oncol Biol Phys 1995;33:809–14.
22. Morgan TO, Jacobsen SJ, McCarthy WF, Jacobsen DJ, McLeod DG, Moul JW. Age-specific reference ranges for prostate-specific antigen in black men. N Engl J Med 1996;335:304–10.
23. Zhu L, Leinonen J, Zhang W-M, Finne P, Stenman UH. Dual-label immunoassay for simultaneous measurement of prostate-specific antigen (PSA)-α1-antichymotrypsin complex together with free or total PSA. Clin Chem 2003;49:97–103.
24. Tunstall-Pedoe H, Kuulasmaa K, Amouyel P, Arveiler D, Rajakangas AM, Pajak A. Myocardial infarction and coronary deaths in the World Health Organization MONICA project. Circulation 1994;90:538–612.
25. Coudrey L. The troponin. Arch Intern Med 1998;158:1173–80.
26. Antman EM, Tanasijevic MJ, Thompson B, Schactman M, McCabe CH, Cannon CP, et al. Cardiac specific troponin I levels to predict the risk of mortality in patients with acute coronary syndromes. N Engl J Med 1996;335:1342–9.
27. Lindahl B, Venge P, Wallentin L, for FRISC study group. Relation between troponin T and the risk of subsequent cardiac events in unstable coronary artery disease. Circulation 1996;93:1651–7.
28. Myocardial infarction redefined—a consensus document of the joint European Society of Cardiology/American College of Cardiology committee for the redefinition of myocardial infarction. J Am Coll Cardiol 2000;36:959–69.
29. Bossuyt PM, Reitsma JB, Bruns DE, Gatsonis CA, Glasziou PP, Irwig LM, et al. Toward complete and accurate reporting of studies of diagnostic accuracy: the STARD initiative. Clin Chem 2003;49:1–6.

4

Measures of Outcome

Andrew St. John and Christopher P. Price

Measurement of outcomes is a crucial part of developing and maintaining an evidence base to support the use of laboratory tests. An outcome is the result of a medical intervention and can be defined in terms of health or cost (1). The evaluation of diagnostic tests can be divided into a number of stages as defined by Fryback and Thornbury (2) and sometimes called a hierarchy of evidence (3). In this hierarchy, the stages are designated as various levels of efficacy, ranging from the initial evaluation of technical efficacy, diagnostic accuracy efficacy, diagnostic thinking efficacy, therapeutic efficacy, patient outcome efficacy, and finally societal efficacy.

It is now widely accepted that the efficacy of a diagnostic test refers to its performance under ideal and controlled conditions. These are the conditions under which most traditional test evaluations are performed. The move toward outcome measurement is about determining the performance of a test in a larger population under the normal conditions of clinical practice. This is defined as effectiveness. The distinction between efficacy and effectiveness is shown in a redefined framework for evaluating tests and shown in Table 1 (4). Thus, outcomes whether for the patient or for society as a whole are defined in the Silverstein and Boland (4) framework as therapeutic effectiveness. Systematic reviews of diagnostic tests generally show that many published evaluations contain little evidence of the effectiveness of a diagnostic test (5–7).

PROBLEMS ASSOCIATED WITH MEASURING OUTCOMES OF LABORATORY TESTS

The paucity of literature about diagnostic outcomes contrasts with therapeutics where outcome measurements are integral to the development, regulatory approval, and marketing of new drugs. This lack is partly because demonstrating the outcome of a treatment is clearer in the sense that the patient gets better or does not. Although laboratory tests can be defined as

Table 1
Framework for evaluation of diagnostic tests (4)

Concept	Measure of test impact
Diagnostic efficacy: test results	
Technical efficacy	Sensitivity and specificity
Clinical efficacy	Positive and negative predictive value
	Yield
Diagnostic effectiveness: new diagnoses	
Diagnostic thinking	Prevalence of disease (pretest probability)
Diagnosis	Positive predictive value (posttest probability)
	Diagnostic yield
Therapeutic efficacy: new therapies	
Therapeutic plan	Physician's intended management plan is usually implicit and not often studied
Actual therapy	Proportion of tests resulting in a change in management
	Therapeutic yield
Therapeutic effectiveness: outcomes	
Patient outcomes	Morbidity, mortality, functional outcomes, costs
Societal outcomes	Cost per diagnosis, treatment, outcome
	Cost per year of life
	Cost per quality-adjusted life year (QALY)

interventions, the outcome or medical response that follows is usually quite remote temporally. In addition, the clinical response to a test result is not always consistent; a physician may institute an intervention despite a negative test result or conversely the physician may fail to take any action in response to a positive result. These difficulties require that special consideration be devoted to the design of outcome studies.

Another reason for the lack of evidence to support the use of many diagnostic tests is that it is ethically difficult to perform procedures such as randomized controlled trials of laboratory tests that are already well established in clinical practice, no matter how little evidence there is for their effectiveness. However, the introduction of new testing modalities such as point-of-care testing (POCT) and of new cardiac markers such as troponins provides an opportunity to study outcomes before these tests become entrenched into clinical practice. Consequently, there have been a significant number of studies identifying outcomes in these two areas of laboratory medicine, several of which will be examined in detail.

With the possible exception of glucose, troponin, and some toxicology measurements, few laboratory tests are crucial to the diagnosis and treatment of life-threatening situations, and so studies of tests that measure mortality and morbidity as outcomes may need to extend over many years. This is particularly true in the case of diseases that have a low prevalence. One solution to this problem is the use of surrogate markers but it is important to ensure that the chosen measure is related to the clinical question, particularly in relation to treatment protocols. While it is possible to use HbA_{1C} measurement as a surrogate for normoglycemia, determining a similar outcome measure for the management of euthyroidism is more difficult. One possibility is a study that determines the rates of complications such as osteoporosis through measurement of bone mineral density or bone markers.

Performing outcome studies of tests such as randomized controlled trials over long periods of time can be expensive, not only from the time perspective, but also because of the large sample numbers that are often required. Manufacturers of the tests evaluated in these trials may determine that the potential income from increased sales of the test being evaluated will not exceed the costs of the trials and consequently they will not provide the necessary funds for such studies.

The difficulty associated with the need for large sample numbers can be partly overcome by carrying out smaller randomized controlled trials to a standard design that allows them to be combined in a meta-analysis. The CONSORT statement, originally intended for therapeutic trials, can also be used for trials of laboratory tests (8). Solutions to the problem of inconsistent clinical responses to the result of a test include a study design that ensures that participants agree to a particular course of action, depending upon the result (9). The disadvantage of such a strategy is that it may not reflect what happens in the real world and by itself may introduce bias to the study.

Other problems of conducting studies to measure outcomes of diagnostic tests include masking the participants to the results of the test and the issue of allocation concealment which aims to prevent preferential performance of the test in certain individuals (10).

TYPES OF OUTCOME MEASUREMENTS

There are many different outcome measures described in the literature and they can be classified in a number of different ways with considerable overlap between them. Table 2 shows some of the measures relevant to determining the outcomes of diagnostic tests and specific examples of these from the literature will be discussed in more detail.

Table 2
Types of outcome measures

Type of outcome	Clinical	Operational (applicable to certain types of service delivery)	Economic
Hard	Mortality Morbidity	Time to treatment	Quality-adjusted life year (QALY) Cost of episode Cost of treatment
Surrogate, intermediate, or soft	Disease markers: *urine albumin* *HbA₁C* *bone mineral density* *cholesterol* *BNP* *PSA* *parathormone* *urinary collagen crosslink molecules* *D-dimer*	Length of stay Number of clinic visits Caregivers' time	Length of stay Use of therapeutics
	Complication rate Readmission rate Patient satisfaction Caregiver satisfaction Functional status		Complication rate Readmission rate

Hard Measurements

One group of outcome measurements can be clearly defined as clinical or "hard" measures and they include mortality and morbidity. They are commonly used as the outcomes of trials of therapeutic drugs but are relatively uncommon when assessing the performance of laboratory testing; one exception is the outcomes that follow from measurement of cardiac markers such as troponins (11).

Surrogate or Intermediate Measurements

It is possible to address some of the problems of remoteness between diagnostic procedure and outcome through the use of surrogate, sometimes called intermediate or "softer," outcomes. Surrogate outcomes or markers should meet two basic criteria. First, there should be a statistical relationship between the proposed marker and the clinical outcome. Second, there should be a pathophysiological basis to the relationship between the surrogate marker and the disease (12). The ideal characteristics of surrogate markers are (13):

- There should be a statistical relationship between the proposed marker and the clinical outcome.
- There should be a clear biological relationship between the marker level and disease activity.
- It can be quantified and delivered in a way that is clinically relevant.
- The marker level should be sensitive and specific in relation to risk of outcome, with acceptable predictive values.
- There should be a defined cutoff between normal and abnormal.
- The change in marker level should relate to response to treatment in a way which is interpretable and meaningful, e.g., rapidly in a life-threatening situation.
- It should be amenable to quality control monitoring

The concept was initially developed in relation to drug trials where such markers can reduce the sample size and duration of trials. However, their reputation in this regard has been tarnished in recent times with the discovery that several surrogate markers have not reliably predicted clinical outcome such as in the case of drug treatment of heart failure (12) and the treatment of AIDS (14). Despite this criticism, surrogate measures remain a valuable tool in assessing the outcomes of laboratory testing procedures. Perhaps the best example of a surrogate outcome is glycated hemoglobin (HbA$_{1C}$) which serves as a surrogate marker for assessing the compliance with therapy in diabetic patients.

Other examples of laboratory tests used in this way are shown in Table 2. Cholesterol is another example of a widely used clinical surrogate. In conjunction with drugs such as simvastatin, the lowering of cholesterol has been found to correlate with reductions in major events such as nonfatal heart attack, the need for revascularization, and overall mortality (15). While the selection of surrogate markers to determine outcomes from drug treatment of heart failure has attracted controversy in the past, more recent studies of the measurement of B-type natriuretic peptide (BNP) show that it appears to correlate with disease progression and parallel the reductions in mortality achieved through beta blocker and angiotensin-converting enzyme therapy (16). Therefore, it is likely that BNP will become a surrogate marker of major importance, the utility of which may be further increased through point-of-care testing.

Measurements such as functional status, quality of life, and patient satisfaction have also been defined as softer, surrogate outcomes.

Clinical, Economic, and Operational Measurements

An alternative way to consider different measures of outcome is from their clinical, operational, or economic impact. A classification on this basis is also shown in Table 2. Clinical outcomes are usually but not exclusively patient related and in addition to mortality and morbidity include disability and functionality and softer but important measures such as patient satisfaction.

Economic measures are sometimes defined as societal benefits because an economic measure such as cost per episode of treatment will usually accrue to the health provider and therefore society as a whole. Some typical economic measures are cost per diagnosis or treatment, cost per year of life, and cost per quality-adjusted life year. More details of these measures are given in chapter 9 of this book.

Operational, process, or management outcome measures are particularly important in relation to POCT (17). A number of studies have examined the effect of this type of testing on the process of care for the patient and its potential to lead to clinical and economic benefits. A typical study compares the length of stay (LOS) in hospital for patients who undergo centralized testing and patients who have their testing carried out at the point of care. As will be described later, study design is critical in such studies as also is a willingness to change the process of care on the basis of the evidence provided (18).

EXERCISES AND EXAMPLES OF OUTCOME MEASUREMENT

The use of different outcome measures is illustrated by the following series of questions or exercises, each of which is followed by an example from the literature that attempts to address a similar question.

Exercise 1: What are the clinical questions to be asked when considering the clinical utility of homocysteine measurement as a cardiac risk factor, and what outcome measures would you use when investigating the claims?

Relationship between Troponin Testing and Mortality (11)

This study utilizes a design that is one of the most powerful in terms of assessing outcomes, namely, a meta-analysis or combining the data from several separate studies, all of which used consecutive patients and where the measured outcome was mortality. It provides strong evidence that a positive troponin result is associated with a substantially increased risk of death or myocardial infarction.

The recent introduction of troponin measurements into clinical practice has provided the laboratory profession with an opportunity to carry out studies to determine whether there is any hard evidence for the effectiveness of these tests. While there are many papers in the literature supposedly evaluating these tests, the study design of many of them is biased in various ways that diminishes the value of the evidence. Because myocardial infarction is a potentially fatal condition, the time span between testing and mortality can be quite short. Consequently, this is one of the relatively uncommon situations where mortality can be measured as the outcome of the test. In other studies which have investigated cardiac markers for risk stratification, indices of morbidity such as chest pain as well as cardiac death have been used as outcome measures.

The study of Heidenreich et al. (11) provides a meta-analysis of data from seven clinical trials and 19 cohort studies which measured troponin levels in a total of 13,000 patients with suspected myocardial infarction but without ST-elevations. The outcomes of this study are shown in Table 3.

Rates of death were approximately 1.5% with a negative troponin test and 6% with a positive result. Negative results occurred in 6% of patients who had the outcomes of death or myocardial infarction while positive results occurred in 16% of the patients.

Table 3
Outcomes in patients suspected of myocardial infarction and undergoing troponin testing

| Test and outcome | Number/total (%) | | Relative risk (95% CI) |
	Positive test	Negative test	
Troponin T			
Death	99/1635 (6.1)	53/3524 (1.5)	4.1 (2.9–5.7)
Death or MI	143/872 (16.4)	85/1412 (6.0)	3.0 (2.3–3.9)
Troponin I			
Death	108/1981 (5.5)	77/4422 (1.7)	3.3 (2.5–4.4)
Death or MI	13/51 (25.5)	12/240 (5.0)	4.9 (2.4–10)

Exercise 2: What outcome measures would you consider when investigating the clinical utility of a POCT service for B-type natriuretic peptide to guide therapy in a heart failure clinic?

Increased Patient Satisfaction through Point-of-Care HbA$_{1C}$ Testing (19)

Grieve et al. (19) compared both patient and nurse satisfaction in two cohorts of patients who used two different modes of service delivery for the surrogate marker HbA$_{1C}$. While patient satisfaction is a softer outcome, it can be measured and it is an important one to the extent that it may influence compliance with treatment as shown in this study.

The U.S. Diabetes Control and Complications Trial (20) and the U.K. Prospective Diabetes Study Group (21) clearly demonstrated the importance of glycemic control in reducing complications and the use of HbA$_{1C}$ as a surrogate marker of glycemia to assist with achieving this goal.

Since these publications, a number of other studies have looked in more detail at the role of POCT or near-patient testing (NPT) in providing HbA$_{1C}$ measurements. Grieve et al. (19) examined the outcome of patient satisfaction in two groups of diabetics, one receiving their HbA$_{1C}$ result at the time of consultation with their doctor (NPT or POCT group), the other obtaining their result later from a central laboratory (conventional testing). The conclusions from their study, which was conducted through questionnaires, were that patients who were in the POCT group were significantly more satisfied with the test information provided than those who were conventionally tested.

Outcomes from this study also included feedback from nurses who had a greater sense of satisfaction with the care process in the POCT group and physicians being able to make more informed decisions when they had immediate access to results through POCT. Moreover patients in the POCT group had a significantly lower HbA$_{1C}$ result compared to the conventional testing group. Similar clinical outcomes have been demonstrated in a randomized control trial of HbA$_{1C}$ by POCT and conventional laboratory testing (22).

Exercise 3: *What study design would you propose, and what outcome measures would you include, to investigate the clinical utility of a POCT service for anticonvulsant drugs?*

Clinical and Economic Outcomes from Monitoring Aminoglycoside Levels in Hematological Malignancies (23)

This study determined economic outcomes from measurement of drug levels in a prospective study of consecutive patients with malignancy and infection. The study results are significant in showing substantial savings if patients are treated on the basis of their therapeutic drug monitoring results but the results will need to be confirmed in a larger group of patients possibly using a different study design.

Much of the literature on therapeutic drug monitoring (TDM) has been criticized as being focused on technical assessment rather than clinical performance and a call has been made for more studies of patient-centered outcomes such as reducing the rate of drug-induced toxicity and improving the success rate of treatment (24). An exception to this situation is the study by Patsalos et al. (25) which showed that epilepsy patients who received their phenytoin results at the time of the consultation achieved optimization of their therapy in a shorter period of time and had less clinic visits compared to those who received their results at a later time.

The study by Binder et al. (23) also addresses past deficiencies through an assessment of the clinical and economic significance of peak aminoglycoside concentrations in patients with fever, neutropenia, and hematological malignancies. The prospective study included 61 consecutive patients who entered a strict treatment protocol for 3 days involving treatment with various antibiotics, followed by a change in treatment for nonresponders. Samples for peak aminoglycoside levels after 3 days of treatment were collected by an independent controller and the results not revealed to the treating clinician.

The results of the study showed a significant dependence of clinical outcome on peak aminoglycoside concentration; 12 of 17 patients with peak concentrations greater than 4.8 mg/L (>10.2 µmol/L) but only 13 of 44 patients with peak concentrations less than or equal to 4.8 mg/L (≤10.2 µmol/L) responded to therapy. The economic outcomes in terms of infection related costs are shown in Table 4. The cost of treating those patients with aminoglycoside levels less than or equal to 4.8 mg/L (≤10.2 µmol/L) were 1.8 times higher than those for levels greater than 4.8 mg/L (>10.2 µmol/L). The total potential savings were calculated to be $167,112 (at 1998 prices).

Table 4
Average patient infection-related costs in U.S. dollars ($US) according to peak aminoglycoside concentration

Costs ($US)	Peak aminoglycoside concentration		Cost difference
	≤4.8mg/L (≤10.2 µmol/L)	>4.8mg/L (>10.2 µmol/L)	
Nursing			
During antibiotic therapy	$1965	$1215	$750
Until discharge	$2576	$1429	$1147
Diagnostics	$2871	$1790	$1081
Therapeutics	$3271	$1701	$1570
Total	$8718	$4920	$3798

Exercise 4: *What are the changes in clinical practice that might be required to achieve the potential economic benefits of providing a new service for troponin measurement?*

Impact of Troponin Determinations on Cost of Care (26)

Zarich et al. (26) used the next best study design after a meta-analysis, that is, a randomized controlled trial to assess health economic outcomes. Other key features of this study include showing that while the laboratory costs of troponin tests are higher than other cardiac markers, this is more than offset by the economic savings related to clinical care. Thus, the clinical outcomes of Heidenreich et al. (11) are supplemented by the economic evidence from this study.

The study population comprised 856 consecutive patients presenting to the emergency department with suspected myocardial infarction who were randomized to receive a standard evaluation of serial ECG and creatine kinase MB isoenzyme (CKMB) tests (control group) or the same tests plus troponin T (troponin group). These tests were undertaken at presentation and at 3 and 12 hours after presentation. The main outcome measurements were length of stay and hospital charges. A prespecified subgroup analysis divided the patients into those with and without acute coronary syndrome. The final diagnosis was made by a cardiologist who was not aware of the troponin values.

The key outcomes (Table 5) were that length of stay was significantly shorter for patients who had troponin measurements in groups of patients in whom acute coronary syndrome was either ruled in or ruled out. Hospital charges were less for both groups but significantly so for those with acute coronary syndrome.

In addition to the significant economic outcomes from this well-designed study, it is also possible to calculate from the data in the paper that the posttest probability of a myocardial infarction with a positive troponin test was about 45%. In other words, a positive test is extremely good at *ruling in* the diagnosis of myocardial infarction.

Exercise 5: *How would you design a study to investigate the clinical utility of urinalysis for leucocyte esterase, nitrite, and protein for the "detection" of urinary tract infection, and what outcome measures would you use?*

Reductions in Laboratory Costs through Use of a Point-of-Care Test for C-Reactive Protein in General Practice (27)

On the basis of previous evidence, Dahler-Eriksen et al. (27) set out to demonstrate both improved clinical and economic outcomes of providing more

Table 5
Key outcomes in a randomized trial of diagnostic strategies for diagnosis of myocardial infarction

Diagnosis	Outcome	Control group	Troponin group	P value
Acute coronary syndrome ruled out (*n* = 654)	Length of stay, days	1.6 ± 3.4	1.2 ± 2.9	0.03
	Hospital charges	$6187 ± 11,256	$4487 ± 7396	0.17
Acute coronary syndrome (*n* = 202)	Length of stay, days	4.6 ± 3.6	3.7 ± 3.2	0.01
	Hospital charges	$19,202 ± 15,933	$15,004 ± 15,277	0.02

rapid C-reactive protein (CRP) results using a randomized crossover trial design of consecutive patients. The study showed substantial cost savings but clinical benefits from less antibiotic prescriptions could not be demonstrated. However, the authors identified the key issues of lack of education and guidelines as possible reasons for not attaining the desired clinical outcomes of the study.

Point-of-care CRP measurements can be used in general practice to differentiate between bacterial and viral infections and provide better guidance on the prescription of antibiotics than can be obtained from measurement of the erythrocyte sedimentation rate (ESR) (28). Dahler-Eriksen et al. (27) determined the economic outcomes from doing this test in the office compared to sending the test to a hospital laboratory. Potential savings could accrue from a number of outcomes, including less prescribing of antibiotics but also less utilization of other laboratory tests such as ESR.

The study design was a randomized crossover trial operating in 29 general practice clinics where the clinics were randomized into two groups; one used a near-patient test (NPT) for CRP while the other mailed CRP samples to a hospital laboratory. After 3 months, there was a crossover of the two groups and the trial proceeded for another 4 months. A total of 1853 patients was recruited into the study. The various outcomes are shown in Table 6.

Although this study is cited primarily for its economic outcome, it also demonstrated operational outcomes that can be achieved by changes to ser-

Table 6
Key outcomes from use of CRP at point of care

Outcome	Result	Statistical significance
Use of ESR tests	Decrease in NPT group of 8%	95% CI (1–14%)
Samples mailed to laboratory	Decrease in NPT group of 6%	95% CI (1–10%)
Changes in prescription of antibiotics	No reduction	
Patients requiring follow-up telephone calls	Reduction from 63% in control group to 53% in NPT group	$P = 0.0001$
Time period for starting of antibiotics in patients with CRP >5.0 mg/dL (>50 mg/L)	Started earlier in NPT group	$P = 0.0161$
Savings per year	$111,160 per year per 340,000 people	

vice provision using POCT. From an economic perspective, the savings that resulted were modest and accrued primarily from reduction in testing by the central laboratory. However, it is important to note that net savings were achieved, despite the fact that the CRP test carried out in the office is more expensive than the one measured by the central laboratory. By examining the whole process and taking into account all of the changes that might result from using POCT, it is possible to achieve a reduction in overall costs.

The cost savings from this study would have been greater if changes to antibiotic prescription had been achieved but this was not the case. The authors argue cogently for the dissemination of clinical guidelines that include predictive values for CRP at key decision levels as a way to improve antibiotic utilization.

Exercise 6: What outcome measures would you utilize when designing a study to determine the clinical utility of the measurement of procalcitonin for the detection of sepsis in a critically ill patient?

Reductions in Use of Blood Products through Use of a Point-of-Care Hemostasis System in Open-Heart Surgery Patients (29)

Despotis et al. (29) demonstrated the significant economic outcomes which result from using less therapeutic products. This is achieved by providing timely coagulation results by POCT during open-heart surgery. The study design was prospective with patients randomized to a control or intervention cohort; it is not stated whether patients were consecutive and, if not, this may be a source of bias. Several other studies have shown economic benefits from timely anticoagulant monitoring but further data are required to demonstrate improved clinical outcomes.

A number of outcome-related studies have been carried out in the area of coagulation monitoring and patients undergoing open-heart surgery. Once again the studies involve the use of handheld devices or POCT to provide more rapid results, which can facilitate decisions about more guided therapy. Postoperative blood loss is a common complication of open-heart surgery, due to a number of factors including hemostasis abnormalities. Treatment for this condition is largely empirical based on results provided by the central laboratory, which is not timely enough to allow more tailored therapy for individual patients.

Despotis et al. (29) carried out a prospective cohort study where patients were randomized to a control or an intervention group. The control group received a fixed anticoagulation protocol treatment regime following bypass while the intervention group received anticoagulation and protamine therapy based on using results from the point-of-care hemostasis testing system.

Compared to the intervention group, the patients in the control group showed the following economic and clinical-based outcomes:

- They received substantially less platelets, fresh frozen plasma, and cryoprecipitate.
- They had shorter operating times.
- They had less chest drainage in the hours after surgery.

Aside from the economic savings from reduced use of therapeutic products in the intervention group—up to $250,000 per annum (at 1997 prices) in this instance—there was also the possibility of additional savings from patients spending less time in high-dependency care.

Exercise 7: What are the clinical presentations that warrant the use of POCT in the emergency room and what outcome measures would you utilize in order to demonstrate an operational benefit?

Randomized Controlled Trials of POCT in Emergency Departments (30, 31)

These two studies represent the best in terms of study design in that both are randomized controlled trials that assessed similar outcomes but produced somewhat different results. In one, there was no difference in outcome, but in the other, POCT patients had a reduced length of stay. Perhaps most importantly, both studies offer some insight into the complexity of care in an emergency department, the difficulty of teasing out which processes can be changed in order to produce improved outcomes, and how to ensure compliance with the study design.

The application of POCT in the emergency room or department has been the subject of several studies in addition to the two discussed here (32–34). While there is no argument that POCT can reduce turnaround times, provide quicker results, and even reduce the time for decision making in some cases, its effect on patient outcomes such as length of stay has been more difficult to document.

The study by Kendall et al. (30) randomized 1728 patients to either POCT or central laboratory testing. The POC tests included blood gases and electrolytes. The outcome measures assessed in this trial which are typical of other studies of POCT in the emergency department are:

- Mortality
- Length of stay in hospital
- Admission rates from emergency department
- Amount of time spent waiting for results of blood tests

- Length of stay in emergency department
- Number of times POCT changed diagnosis, treatment plan, or plans for further care
- Number of times POCT brought about time critical changes in treatment

The results showed significantly faster decision making in the POCT group, which produced a time-critical benefit in 6.9% of patients while POCT influenced treatment in 14% of cases overall. There were no major differences between the groups in the other outcomes listed such as mortality and length of stay. The reasons for the lack of impact on length of stay was believed to be due to the fact that the availability of blood tests was not the rate-limiting step but issues such as bed availability were likely to be more important.

The study by Murray et al. (31) randomized 180 patients to POCT (blood gases, electrolytes, and metabolites) or central laboratory testing. The length of stay (LOS) was the primary measure of outcome. In the POCT group, the median LOS (3 hr 28 min) was significantly reduced compared to the patient tested in the central laboratory (4 hr 22 min). While the study concluded that POCT can achieve significant time savings, this reduction was only apparent in the patients who were sent home.

The overall conclusion from studies of POCT in emergency departments is that the effect on patient outcomes of POCT is marginal at best, primarily because there are other factors that affect the care process. In addition, the different conclusions from the two studies discussed here suggest that the outcomes are significantly dependent upon the circumstances and practices of the institution.

Exercise 8: What tools would you use in order to identify the need for a change in procedures in order to maximize the benefit from POCT, and how would you implement change?

Prospective Application of POCT to Improve Patient Waiting Time (35)

The study of Nichols et al. (35) provides a model example of how to take advantage of the benefits offered by POCT and provide a better outcome in the form of improved patient satisfaction. The study was a before-and-after design and like the studies of POCT in the emergency departments, the complexity of the care process is highlighted. However, in this study, the authors could identify and make changes to the process and thereby achieve their goals.

The main goal of this study was to reduce the patient waiting time for interventional procedures which required laboratory testing beforehand. Thus, the primary outcome was one of patient satisfaction.

They prospectively studied 217 patients over a 7-month period in a number of distinct phases. Phase 1 was a workflow analysis, followed by implementation of POCT in phase 2 for renal and coagulation parameters in parallel with central laboratory testing. Full implementation of POCT took place in phase 3 where significant reductions in waiting time occurred for renal testing compared to the central laboratory but not for coagulation testing.

Following changes to the process of clinical management which resulted in a more complete integration of POCT into the cardiovascular laboratory, phase 4 showed significantly reduced waiting times also for coagulation testing. The reductions in waiting time for renal testing were also maintained in the latter phase.

This study, like those is the emergency room discussed earlier, highlights the fact that provision of faster testing, although important by itself in certain circumstances, is not always the rate-limiting step. In the circumstances of this study, it was possible for the authors to make changes to the process and then reassess the effects of their changes. Clearly, the complexity of some care processes such as in emergency departments does not always make this approach possible. However, it is important to realize that simply changing the way testing is delivered may not always yield the desired outcomes.

SUMMARY

The design of studies to demonstrate the benefits associated with the use of a diagnostic test are extremely challenging. A considerable amount of the literature on diagnostic tests has been concerned with the science relating the test to the pathophysiology of the disease and with the analytical methods associated with the measurement of the marker. Furthermore, most of the data on diagnostic test results in the clinical situation has been developed "in parallel" with the clinical care of the patient, rather than being used to guide the management of the patient. Consequently, little data identifies a pivotal role for the test, although observational studies and clinical audit projects have shown how important the test result can be (36).

The diagnostic test provides only one piece of the information that is used to make a clinical decision, and consequently designing a study which identifies that unique role can be very difficult. Indeed, the design of a study that focuses on one element of a multifaceted process can lead to a study protocol that does not match the current standard of clinical practice. Thus, when Coster et al. (37) found little evidence from randomized controlled trials to support the frequent use of blood glucose monitoring in type 2 diabetes, they had to question the conclusions as most of the studies had not taken account of the important role of education in diabetes management.

However, as has been pointed out in this chapter, there is the risk of bias in the results when studies seek to ensure compliance with a specific protocol encompassing several potential variables.

Despite these limitations, there is a clear need to find a study design that can help to identify the role of a diagnostic test, especially as new tests and testing modalities continue to be released. The key features of the study design have to test whether access to the test result leads to an improvement in health outcome for the patient (38); some examples have been illustrated in this chapter, although study design for diagnostic tests is still a controversial area (9).

A crucial feature of the study is the outcome measure against which the use of the test is judged. While morbidity and mortality are the primary outcome indices, it is obvious that there are many limitations to their use. First, in many situations the studies take a long time to reach these endpoints. Second, there are so many elements of the "clinical process" that will impact upon these outcome measures that it would be difficult to judge the contribution made by the diagnostic test. Consequently, the use of a surrogate endpoint provides a more practical solution.

It has to be demonstrated that a surrogate clinical endpoint measure relates to the pathophysiology of the disease. Changes in the surrogate marker must show a close correlation to changes in the activity of the disease, and it must be possible to quantify the marker accurately and precisely. The marker may be related to the disease process or to a complication of the disease, and there must be evidence to support this relationship.

The economic measures in many respects also require the identification of a number of perspectives. Thus, one might take a societal view on the benefit from using a test; however, a shorter term perspective is required both in terms of the practicality of measurement of the benefit, as well as in being able to make use of the information in policy making. Thus, it is easier to measure the changes in utilization of resources, such as blood products, other testing modalities, and staff, as well as the length of stay than it is to assess the cost per episode and years of life gained. More importantly, it is possible to translate these measures into actions that might need to be taken to change practice and deliver economic benefits in the short term.

Identifying outcome measures that can be quantified is therefore important in order to demonstrate the potential value of a test. These outcome measures can also help to point to the way in which practice may need to be modified in order to deliver the real clinical and economic benefits.

REFERENCES

1. Bissell MG. Laboratory related measures of patient outcomes: an introduction. Washington: AACC Press, 200:194 pp.

2. Fryback FG, Thornbury JR. The efficacy of diagnostic imaging. Med Decis Making 1991;11:88–94.

3. Pearl WS. A hierarchical outcomes approach to test assessment. Ann Emerg Med 1999;33:77–84.

4. Silverstein MD, Boland BJ. Conceptual framework for evaluating laboratory tests: case-finding in ambulatory patients. Clin Chem 1994;40:1621–7.

5. Hobbs FDR, Delaney BC, Fitzmaurice DA, Wilson S, Hyde CJ, Thorpe GH, et al. A review of near patient testing in primary care. Health Technol Assess 1997;1:1–230.

6. Balk EM, Ioannidis JP, Salem D, Chew PW, Lau J. Accuracy of biomarkers to diagnose acute cardiac ischemia in the emergency department: a meta-analysis. Ann Emerg Med 2001;37:478–94.

7. Gorelich MH, Shaw KN. Screening tests for urinary tract infection. Pediatrics 1999;104:1–7.

8. Begg C, Cho M, Eastwood S, Horton R, Moher D, Olkin I, et al. Improving the quality of reporting of randomized controlled trials. The CONSORT statement. J Am Med Assoc 1996;276:637–9.

9. Bossuyt PMM, Lijmer JG, Mol BWJ. Randomised comparisons of medical tests: sometimes invalid, not always efficient. Lancet 2000;356:1844–7.

10. Bruns DE. Laboratory-related outcomes in healthcare. Clin Chem 2001;47:1547–52.

11. Heidenreich PA, Alloggiamento T, Melsop K, McDonald KM, Go AS, Hlatky MA. The prognostic value of troponin in patients with non-ST elevation acute coronary syndromes: a meta-analysis. J Am Coll Cardiol 2001;38:478–85.

12. Lipicky RJ, Packer M. Role of surrogate end points in the evaluation of drugs of heart failure. J Am Coll Cardiol 1993;22:Suppl A,179A–84A.

13. Greenhalgh T. Surrogate endpoints. In: How to read a paper: the basics of evidence based medicine. 2nd ed. London: BMJ Publishing Group, 2001:97–101.

14. Jacobson MA, Bacchetti P, Kolokathis A, Chaisson RE, Szabo S, Polsky B, et al. Surrogate markers for survival in patients with AIDS and AIDS related complex treated with zidovudine. Br Med J 1991;302:73–8.

15. Scandinavian Simvastatin Survival Study Group. Randomised trial of cholesterol lowering in 4444 patients with coronary heart disease: the Scandinavian Simvastatin Survival Study. Lancet 1994;344:1389–99.

16. Lee CR, Adams KF Jr, Patterson JH. Surrogate end points in heart failure. Ann Pharmacother 2002;36:479–88.

17. Rainey PM. Outcomes assessment for point of care testing. Clin Chem 1998;44:1595–6.

18. Price CP. Point of care testing: potential for tracking disease management outcomes. Dis Manage Health Outcomes 2002;10:749–61.

19. Grieve R, Beech R, Vincent J, Mazurkiewicz J. Near patient testing in diabetes clinics: appraising the costs and outcomes. Health Technol Assess 1999;3;1–74.

20. Diabetes Control and Complications Trial Research Group. Lifetime benefits and costs of intensive therapy as practiced in the Diabetes Control and Complications Trial. J Am Med Assoc 1996;276:1409–15.

21. Gray A, Raikou M, McGuire A, Fenn P, Stevens R, Cull C, et al. Cost effectiveness of an intensive blood glucose control policy in patients with type 2 diabetes: economic analysis alongside randomised controlled trail (UKPDS 41). Br Med J 2000;320:1373–8.

22. Cagliero E, Levina EV, Nathan DM. Immediate feedback of HbA1C levels improves glycaemic control in type 1 and insulin-treated type 2 diabetic patients. Diabetes Care 1999;22:1785–9.

23. Binder L, Schiel X, Binder C, Menke CF, Schuttrumpf S, Armstrong VW, et al. Clinical outcome and economic impact of aminoglycoside peak concentrations in febrile immunocompromised patients with hematologic malignancies. Clin Chem 1998;44:408–14.

24. Schumacher GE, Barr JT. Total testing process applied to therapeutic drug monitoring: impact on patients' outcomes and economics. Clin Chem 1998;44:370–4.

25. Patsalos PN, Sander JWAS, Oxley J. Immediate anticonvulsant drug monitoring in management of epilepsy. Lancet 1987;2:39.

26. Zarich S, Bradley K, Seymour J, Ghah W, Traboulsi A, Mayall ID, et al. Impact of troponin T determinations of hospital resource utilization and costs in the evaluation of patients with suspected myocardial ischemia. Am J Cardiol 2001;88:732–6.

27. Dahler-Eriksen BS, Lauritzen T, Lassen JF, Lund ED, Brandslund I. Near-patient test for C-reactive protein in general practice: assessment of clinical, organizational and economic outcomes. Clin Chem 1999;45:478–85.

28. Hansson LO, Carlsson I, Hansson E, Hovelius B, Svensson P, Tryding N. Measurement of C-reactive protein and the erythrocyte sedimentation rate in general practice. Scand J Prim Health Care 1995;13:39–45.

29. Despotis GJ, Joist JH, Goodnough LT. Monitoring of hemostasis in cardiac surgical patients: impact of point of care testing on blood loss and transfusion outcomes. Clin Chem 1997;43:1684–7.

30. Kendall J, Reeves B, Clancy M. Point of care testing: randomized controlled trial of clinical outcome. Br Med J 1998;316:1052–7.

31. Murray RP, Leroux M, Sabga E, Palatnick W, Ludwig L. Effect of point of care testing on length of stay in an adult emergency department. J Emerg Med 1999;17:811–4.

32. Saxena S, Wong S. Does the emergency room need a dedicated stat laboratory? Continuous quality improvement as a management tool for the clinical laboratory. Am J Clin Pathol 1993;100:606–10.

33. Parvin CA, Lo SF, Deuser SM, Weaver LG, Lewis LM, Scott MG. Impact of point of care testing on patient's length of stay in a large emergency department. Clin Chem 1996;42:711–7.

34. van Heyningen C, Watson ID, Morrice AE. Point-of-care testing outcomes in an emergency department. Clin Chem 1999;45:437–8.

35. Nichols JH, Kickler TS, Dyer K, Humbertson SK, Cooper PC, Maughan WL, et al. Clinical outcomes of point-of-care testing in the interventional radiology and invasive cardiology setting. Clin Chem 2000; 46:543–50.

36. Karter AJ, Ackerson L, Darbinian JA, D'Agostino RB Jr, Ferrara A, Liu J, et

al. Self-monitoring of blood glucose levels and glycemic control: the Northern California Kaiser Permanente Diabetes registry. Am J Med 2001;111:1–9.

37. Coster S, Gulliford MC, Seed PT, Powrie JK, Swaminathan R. Monitoring blood glucose in diabetes mellitus: a systematic review. Health Tech Assess 2000;4:1–93.

38. Sackett DL, Haines RB, The architecture of diagnostic research. Br Med J 2002;321:539–41.

5

Study Design and Quality of Evidence

Patrick M.M. Bossuyt

The evaluation of medical tests differs substantially from the way in which pharmaceutical products are studied. The evidence for diagnostic tests is rarely adequately evaluated before tests enter common clinical use. There are no international standards of assessment, and little methodological research has been undertaken to systematically evaluate, promote, and develop new or existing technology.

At present, evaluating the effectiveness of medical tests is centered around studies of reproducibility and diagnostic accuracy. In studies of diagnostic accuracy, results from one or more tests are compared with the results obtained with the reference standard on the same subjects. Diagnostic accuracy can be expressed in a number of ways, including sensitivity–specificity pairs, likelihood ratios, diagnostic odds ratios, and areas under receiver operating characteristic (ROC) curves (*see* chapter 7).

For years sensitivity, specificity, and related measures have been described as fixed test characteristics. To evaluate a test, all one needed was simply to measure them. There was little or no attention to how these features were quantitatively expressed or to issues of design and statistical uncertainty. As a consequence, issues of variability and applicability received little or no attention in papers reporting diagnostic accuracy.

There is now ample evidence that sensitivity and specificity are not properties of a test itself. They describe the behavior of a test under specific circumstances that have to be identified and well described. Furthermore, it has been demonstrated that poor studies of diagnostic tests can produce biased estimates (1–3). Design does matter, as it does in any form of clinical research or healthcare technology evaluation.

This chapter summarizes current understanding of design differences as sources of bias and lack of applicability. The first part contains a description of diagnostic accuracy studies in which one test is compared with a reference standard. Such studies aim to establish the diagnostic accuracy of the test. The second part discusses comparative diagnostic accuracy studies.

To know the diagnostic accuracy of a single test is important. Good accuracy is a necessary but not sufficient condition to decide whether a test is clinically useful. The user can only be really confident in the value of a test if it is known that availability of the test result leads to more effective healthcare by increasing effectiveness, by resulting in more efficient use of resources, or both. For this reason, the research on medical tests is moving in a different direction that is characterized by the use of comparative designs and an increasing emphasis on improved patient outcome. There will be more comparative studies where testing is compared with no testing and further clinical action has to be based on the available information.

Some of these designs are introduced in the second part of this chapter which covers issues that are more relevant for decision making. Several comparative designs are presented that focus on patient outcome, and issues surrounding randomized trials of medical tests are discussed briefly.

SINGLE DIAGNOSTIC ACCURACY STUDIES

In single studies of diagnostic accuracy, the outcomes from one test are compared with outcomes from the reference standard. Both tests are applied in a series of patients suspected for a particular target condition. Figure 1A shows the basic structure of this study design.

The term "test" refers not just to laboratory tests; a test can be any method for obtaining additional information on a patient's health status. This includes laboratory tests, imaging tests, function tests, and histopathology, as well as data from the patient history, physical examination, and genetic data. There is no fundamental difference between the evaluation of a laboratory test and other tests in healthcare. All tests are used to reduce uncertainty about the presence of the target condition in a patient.

The term "diagnostic accuracy" refers to expressions of the agreement between the information from the index test and the reference standard that is obtained from a cross-classification of the outcomes of the index test and the results of the reference standard. Diagnostic accuracy can be expressed in many ways, including sensitivity and specificity, likelihood ratios, diagnostic odds ratio, and the area under a ROC curve. These concepts and methods as well as their application are discussed in detail in chapters 7 and 8.

There are several potential threats to the internal and external validity of a study of diagnostic accuracy. Poor internal validity will produce bias, or systematic error, because the estimates do not correspond to what one would have obtained using optimal methods. Poor external validity limits the generalizability of the findings. In that case, the results of the study, even if unbiased, do not correspond to the data needs of the deci-

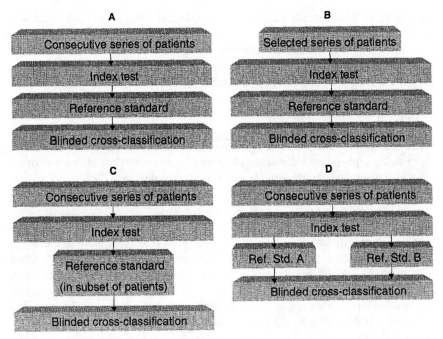

Figure 1   Diagnostic accuracy studies.

A: Basic design for a diagnostic accuracy study (e.g., a cohort design strategy) .

B: Selection: not all consecutive patients are invited to the study. High risk of spectrum or selection bias results from this strategy.

C: Partial verification: not all test results are verified by the reference standard. This strategy represents a form of verification bias.

D: Differential verification: test results are verified by two or more reference standards. This strategy represents a form of verification bias.

sion-maker. The most important sources of bias and lack of applicability will now be addressed.

Selection of Patients

As measures of diagnostic accuracy express the behavior of a test under particular circumstances, test behavior will differ, depending on the group or population of patients that undergoes testing. Test evaluations should therefore include an appropriate spectrum of patients in whom the target condition is suspected in clinical practice, in other words the patient group in whom the clinical question is being asked, specifying the amount of prior testing these patients have received. The ideal study examines a consecutive series of patients, enrolling all consenting patients suspected of the target condition within a specific period. All of these patients then undergo the index test and then the reference test. This resembles the cohort design as it is known in epidemiology.

The term "consecutive" is so misused in the literature that it has almost lost its meaning. The term refers to total absence of any form of selection beyond the a priori definition of the criteria for inclusion and exclusion and explicit efforts to identify patients qualifying for inclusion. Not enrolling consecutive patients can lead to spectrum or selection bias (4) (Figure 1B).

Alternative designs are possible, some of which can be quite difficult to unravel. Some studies first select patients known to have the target condition and then contrast the results of these patients with those from a control group. These designs are similar to case-control designs.

As in any case-control design, the selection of the control group is critical. If the control group consists of only healthy individuals, diagnostic accuracy of the test will be overestimated. In practice, patients suspected for the target condition who test negative with the reference standard usually have other signs, complaints, and conditions that prompted the ordering of the tests. These conditions can produce false-positive results. In contrast, healthy volunteers are usually without such complaints and are less likely to obtain false-positive results. In quantitative terms, the mean of the distributions of test results of healthy controls will be well separated from those of patients with the target condition.

Case-control designs are frequently used in the early phases of test evaluation at which time researchers look at a group of patients known to have the disease and a group of people who definitely are known not to have it, rather than patients merely suspected of having it (5, 6).

Case-control designs, however, do not always lead to optimistic impressions of diagnostic accuracy. If the control group consists of patients with established diagnoses, which differ from but are related to the target condition, making a distinction between cases and controls can become quite a challenge, maybe even more difficult than in clinical practice. In this situation, diagnostic accuracy will be underestimated.

The setting of the diagnostic accuracy study and the associated referral pattern of patients can also affect estimates of diagnostic accuracy. A test would be expected to perform better in populations with more severe disease, as this is generally easier to detect than mild disease. In reality, the distributions of test results differ from setting to setting. They are not identical in primary care versus secondary care, where typically only more advanced cases will be seen.

Reference Standard

The diagnostic accuracy paradigm is based on comparisons of the outcomes of the test under study with those from the reference standard. Originally, the paradigm relied on a quest for the gold standard, a search for the ideal measure to establish the "true disease status" of the patient. However, the concept of a gold standard is as elusive as the holy grail. For many conditions, there simply is no gold standard, the gold standard is rusty, or it is unavailable. Furthermore, for a wide range of conditions, the gold standard does not offer the most meaningful way of defining the target condition, because the circumstances that define meaningful also advance clinical action.

Pulmonary embolism offers a good example of the difficulties associated with the gold standard discussion (7). One gold standard has been the use of autopsy data, but these are not always available: most patients with pulmonary embolism do not die and not all that do expire have an autopsy performed. As an alternative, the use of clinical assessment has been proposed. That concept is quite simple: monitor patients with negative study findings to see how they do. In practice, this approach can be difficult because patients with a strong suspicion of pulmonary embolism will receive treatment. Thus, one would expect fewer recurrences within treated test-positive patients compared to test-negative patients. Egermayer (8) reviewed available data regarding the followup of patients with pulmonary embolism who were untreated. The two studies he found reported disturbingly high recurrence rates in treated compared to untreated groups.

In the framework used in this chapter, the reference standard is the best available method for establishing the presence or absence of the target condition. The reference standard can be either a single procedure or a combination of methods that may include laboratory tests, imaging tests, pathology, as well as dedicated clinical followup of subjects. Combinations are known as composite reference standards.

The reliability of reference standards can be variable; less reliable reference standards lead to misclassification of patients and underestimation of test accuracy, particularly if the reference standard and test are uncorrelated. Reference test error bias occurs when errors of imperfect reference standards bias the measurement of diagnostic accuracy of the index test.

The reference standard may not always be applied to all patients tested with the index test. This may happen if the reference standard is an invasive procedure, but it could also be due to negligence or other factors. If not all patients are verified with the reference standard, verification bias may occur. Two forms of verification bias exist: partial verification bias and differential verification bias (9–12).

Partial verification applies when not all patients are tested. It will lead to bias if the selection is not purely random but associated with the outcome of the index test and the strength of prior suspicion. Partial verification can be the outcome of workup bias, when patients with positive or negative diagnostic test results are preferentially referred to receive verification of diagnosis by the reference standard procedure.

Figure 1C offers a schematic description of partial verification. In a typical case, test negatives are not verified by the invasive reference standard, resulting in underestimation of the number of false negatives. A statistical fix has been proposed to solve this problem (10), but one can question the applicability of this strategy, given the many fundamental assumptions of this approach and the limited number of patients in a typical diagnostic study.

Even if all patients are verified, a different form of verification bias can happen if more than one reference standard is used, and the two reference standards correspond to different manifestations of disease. This can give rise to differential verification bias (Figure 1D). For instance, suppose test-positive patients are verified with further testing, while test-negative patients are verified by clinical followup. An example is the verification of suspected appendicitis with histopathology of the appendix versus natural history as two components of the reference standard. A patient is counted as a false positive if the additional test does not confirm the presence of disease after a positive index test. Alternatively, a patient is classified as a false negative if an event is observed during followup after a negative test result. Yet these are different definitions of disease because not all pathology-positive patients will experience an event during followup if left untreated. Due to the ambiguous definition of disease, with one definition close to pathology and a second closer to clinical prognosis, differential verification will cause a distorted view of test properties and performance.

The timing of the reference standard can be critical. Larger intervals between test and verification by the reference standard may lead to disease progression bias. In that case, the disease is at a more advanced stage when the reference standard is performed and clear cases appear to have been missed by the index test, whereas they were not detectable at the time that index testing had been performed. As the time interval grows larger, the actual condition of the patient may change, leading to more expressed forms of the alternative conditions.

In fact, anything that happens between administration of the index test and the reference test can affect the estimates of diagnostic accuracy. In clinical practice, index test positive patients are likely to be treated, if such treatment is available. If treatment is started before the results are verified by the reference standard, if that treatment is effective, and if the condition responds rapidly to such treatment, then it may be difficult to establish the true status of these patients, leading to the treatment paradox. Index test (true) positives can convert to negative on the reference standard, even if they originally corresponded to true disease. An example is the rapid use of antibiotics in suspected bacterial infection and the use of culture as a reference standard.

Review bias occurs when interpretation of the index test or reference standard is influenced by knowledge of the results of the other test. Diagnostic review bias occurs when the results of the index test are known while interpreting the reference standard. Analogously, test review bias can be present when outcomes of the reference standard are known while interpreting the index test.

In some cases, it may be inevitable or preferable to use a panel to assign a final diagnosis, and to disclose the index test results to that panel, in addition to data on followup and other procedures. When the result of the index test is used in establishing the final diagnosis, incorporation bias may occur. This incorporation will probably increase the amount of agreement between index test results and the outcome of the reference standard, and hence this step overestimates the various measures of diagnostic accuracy. In that case, agreement between the index test and the reference standard—the judgment of the panel—can be artificially inflated, leading to biased estimates of diagnostic accuracy.

There is a long-standing debate on whether or not clinical data should be provided to those reading the index test when that test has a subjective component (13). Withholding that information is known as blinding or masking. For most study questions, masking is preferable. Interpreters are also more likely to consider results from (subjective) tests abnormal in settings with higher prevalence. This tendency is known as context bias (14).

Analysis

In many cases, the results of a diagnostic accuracy study can be summarized using a two-by-two table or, more generally, an n-by-n table. As simple as it seems, the construction of such a table requires special attention. One particular case is the existence of indeterminate results. The frequency of indeterminate results will limit a test's applicability or make it cost more because further diagnostic procedures are needed. Whether bias will arise depends on the association between uninterpretable test results and the target condition.

A second case is the definition of the threshold value, also termed a cutoff or decision point, used to classify test results as either negative or positive. This threshold should be specified prior to the collection of data. This is because selecting post-hoc a cutoff point to maximize the diagnostic accuracy of the test may lead to optimistic measures of test performance. Often the group of patients used to establish the cutoff is termed the training set. Examining the performance of this cutoff in a second independent set of patients termed the test set will almost always be lower, even if the study consists of comparable patients recruited in the same center.

As with all statistical measures, the stability of sensitivity and specificity depends on how many patients have been evaluated. Surprisingly, few studies have taken this fact into account. Like many other measures, any point estimate should be accompanied by confidence intervals around it, which are easily calculated (15).

Variability and Lack of Applicability

The previous subsections summarized the evidence on bias in diagnostic accuracy that can produce a distorted view of the properties of a test due to shortcomings in the way data have been collected and analyzed. Yet even when tests are evaluated in a study with adequate quality—including features such as consecutive patients, a good reference standard, and independent, blinded assessments of tests and the reference standard—diagnostic test performance in one setting may vary from the results reported elsewhere (16). These may represent genuine differences between test accuracy in different settings, such as primary care or in-hospital, different types of hospitals, or the same type of hospital in different countries. Sources of genuine variability are different definitions of disease (i.e., the target condition) and testing procedures. Performance may differ between tests that bear the same generic name but are produced by different manufacturers. D-Dimer tests are an example; less sensitive versions, such as most latex agglutination formats, are intended for screening patients for disseminated intravascular coagulation (DIC); however, more sensitive ELISA-type formats are intended both for DIC screening and assessment of deep vein thrombosis or pulmonary embolism. Despite these clinically important differences in sensitivity, both assay types are generically known as tests for D-dimer. Also, tests may not perform in the same way when produced in kit form, compared to initial laboratory testing in the development phase (17).

Sensitivity and specificity should in general be considered as average values for a population. Diagnostic studies should be large enough to explore the clinical meaning of variability between pertinent individual subgroups within the spectrum of tested patients.

Poor Reporting

The relative magnitude of the different forms of bias is uncertain. One study looked at 26 systematic reviews of diagnostic accuracy studies and compared the outcome in studies with design deficiencies with those without such shortcomings (2). The diagnostic odds ratio in (healthy) case-control studies was threefold higher than in cohort studies examining the same test. Differential verification produced twofold larger diagnostic odds ratios.

The evaluation of evidence from diagnostic test papers is compounded by how poorly they are reported. To remedy this, the Standards for Reporting of Diagnostic Accuracy (STARD) initiative has been started. The objective of the STARD initiative is improvement of the quality of reporting of diagnostic accuracy studies. Following the successful CONSORT initiative to improve the reporting of randomized controlled trials (18), the

STARD initiative aims at the development of a checklist of items that should be included in the report of a study of diagnostic accuracy.

A single-page checklist has been published in the first 2003 issues of several journals including *Annals of Internal Medicine, Radiology, BMJ,* and *Clinical Chemistry* (19). Statement and checklists are accompanied by a separate explanatory document that articulates the meaning and rationale of each item and briefly summarizes the available evidence (20). The documents are also available on several web sites. If medical journals adopt the checklist and the flow diagram, the quality of reporting of studies of diagnostic accuracy should improve to the advantage of clinicians, researchers, reviewers, journals, and the public.

COMPARATIVE DIAGNOSTIC ACCURACY STUDIES

The previous section described the design and analysis of diagnostic accuracy studies. Such data may enable the estimation of parameters such as a test's sensitivity, specificity, and the likelihood ratios corresponding to the respective outcomes of these tests. These parameters can be used in the Bayesian updating of prior probabilities. Yet in other cases, clinicians or healthcare professionals may need comparative data to decide whether they should use one test rather than another. An example is making a choice from the available D-dimer products just mentioned. In that case, decision-makers want to compare the analytical characteristics, diagnostic sensitivities and specificities, or other properties of the tests under consideration.

The basic design of such comparative diagnostic accuracy studies does not differ from the single diagnostic accuracy study discussed earlier. The investigator takes a consecutive series of patients with uncertainty about the target condition, obtains results from both index tests, and verifies them by subjecting all patients to the reference standard.

A major concern in any comparative study is the selection of patients. Whenever the researcher takes any two series of patients, selection bias may occur; the series of patients subjected to the first index test may very well differ from the one for which the second index test is ordered. As a result, any differences in test sensitivity or specificity cannot be reliably attributed solely to the difference in tests. Things may even get worse if different reference standards are used to verify the results of the respective tests, leading to a different form of differential verification bias.

Randomized Designs

There are two ways to circumvent the dangers of selection bias. The straightforward solution is analogous to resolutions used when evaluating therapy; randomization and the use of a common reference standard (Figure 2A). In a randomized comparative diagnostic accuracy study, researchers take consecutive series of consenting patients and use a randomization device—most often a separate computer program—to assign these patients to one index test or a second one. The outcomes of both tests are then verified by comparing them all with the same reference standard.

With such a randomized design, all baseline differences between the two patient groups are compensated for by definition, and any difference exceeding what one would expect based on chance only can be attributed to the difference in tests. Such randomized designs allow for unbiased comparisons and the application of the impressive statistical machinery of experimental design, such as testing for significance and calculating confidence intervals.

Paired Designs

There is a second solution to circumvent selection bias. In therapy trials, it is not possible to study the effects of administering and withholding therapy in the same patients, except in those very rare circumstances where a cross-over design can be used. With questions on diagnosis, paired designs are generally feasible: it is very well possible—at least in principle—to submit the same patient to two tests and compare the outcomes (Figure 2B). Such a paired design relies on a comparison in identical patients and may offer enhanced precision relative to randomized designs.

A paired design cannot be used if the administration of the test would affect the target condition of the test, either directly or indirectly, through

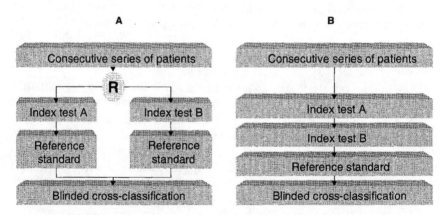

Figure 2 Comparative diagnostic accuracy studies.

A: Randomized comparative diagnostic accuracy study, where R = randomization process using computer or other tool.

B: Paired diagnostic accuracy study

clinical action. It may be considered unethical if the tests to be compared are invasive and/or burdensome procedures. The researcher should also be aware of comparator review bias which occurs when a diagnostic study involves the comparison of two or more diagnostic tests with the reference standard and the results of any of the tests are known when interpreting results.

Before–After Designs

A special form of a paired diagnostic accuracy study is the before–after design. This is a design where one looks at the outcome of one index test, establishes the correspondence between test outcome and the results from the reference standard, and then proceeds to the next index test, the one to be evaluated. The analysis then focuses on the changes in test outcome between the first index test and the second. The before–after design is a simplified form of a comparative design, where one compares the accuracy of one index test only, and the accuracy of that same index test followed by a second test. Knottnerus et al. (21) has offered a more elaborate discussion of this design (22). It must be noted that this design strategy can lead to bias if the first index test has a subjective component. Also, reading a test result can be affected if one knows that a second test is going to be applied anyway. Pretending that no other test is going to follow can be difficult in practice. Thus, the intended behavior may be different from actual behavior.

COMPARATIVE DIAGNOSTIC OUTCOME STUDIES

Diagnostic accuracy is itself important, but not decisive, when making decisions about whether or not to use a specific test. In the end, all healthcare measures will be judged with respect to their ability to maintain or restore a patient's health. Poor accuracy limits the clinical value of a test but, by themselves, high sensitivity and specificity cannot guarantee improvement in patient outcome. In order to determine the true effectiveness of medical tests, the rather intricate ways in which the improvement of health is brought about by medical tests must be considered (*see also* chapter 3).

There are several ways for medical tests to affect a patient's health status. First, undergoing the test itself can have an impact. Few people enjoy having a sample of their blood taken. On the positive side, being tested can have a positive nonspecific effect for patients, regardless the actual test outcome. This is the placebo effect of testing and not that much about the magnitude and modifying factors of these effects is known, other than they exist.

Tests generate information that is infrequently communicated directly to patients. Most often, test information will be used to guide the decisions made by healthcare professionals. These decisions have to do with further testing or other interventions, actions aimed at remedying the patient's complaints or to improve, maintain, or restore their health status. The test result will guide decisions about starting, withholding, modifying, or stopping treatment.

The claim has been made that the most decisive evidence for determining the effectiveness of diagnostic measures should come from randomized comparisons that look at patient outcome rather than diagnostic accuracy (23). This comes as no surprise, as the randomized clinical trial has now become the de facto standard for documenting the effectiveness of all healthcare measures, not just pharmaceuticals. Over the past decades, the randomized clinical trial has evolved from a statistical oddity into the cornerstone of clinical effectiveness research.

Slowly, the number of such randomized outcome trials with diagnostic tests is increasing. Some of the best known studies are the large screening trials, in which one group of patients is invited to participate in a screening program and a control group is not. Patient outcomes in both groups are then compared. These outcomes are influenced both by testing and by further actions guided by the results of testing. Similar trials can be developed for other tests, including imaging and laboratory tests.

There are a number of problems associated with the use of the randomized clinical trial for diagnostic questions that call for caution in designing and interpreting such studies (24). To start, the relation between test and outcome is usually an indirect one. Tests themselves do not usually produce health gains or health hazards, so any randomized design will evaluate both the test and the downstream consequences of testing, including management of other clinical actions. In several trials, the relation between test outcome and further management has been left unspecified, so one cannot distinguish between improper test results and improper subsequent decision making. Furthermore, if treatment is effective, even a random result of a test will produce a difference in patient outcome, making it difficult to attribute differences to quality testing.

Running trials for diagnostic tests without a well-specified protocol for translating the test results to clinical management decisions is analogous to putting pharmaceuticals to trial without prespecifying the preferred dosage, the optimal route of administration, the need for monitoring, or the way to deal with side effects. Designing such a drug trial would be hardly acceptable these days. Why then should the same stringent criteria not be applied to trials of test–treatment combinations?

Trials comparing two tests require large sample sizes that depend on the magnitude of the effect whenever the researcher aims at evaluating differences in patient outcome. To understand the rationale for this claim, consider the simple case of two tests, both used to guide a decision whether or not to treat. The results between the two tests can be expected to show a considerable level of concordance. Many patients will test positive with either test. Differences in outcome between the group using one test and the one using the alternative will be due to chance only. The same applies to patients that would test negative with either test and will not be treated. Here also, any difference will be due to chance only. Therefore, the only group that contributes to the overall difference in outcome is the subgroup with discordant test results. These are the patients that test negative on one test and positive on the other. If treatment is effective, the outcome in this group of patients can be expected to differ, depending on whether one test or the other test is used. It is not difficult to see that the overall differences can be expected to be tiny to small, depending on the level of discordance between the tests and the effectiveness of treatment.

These small overall differences have made researchers wary of studying health outcomes and have caused them to turn to secondary outcome measures, such as length of hospital stay. Although a proper understanding of the use of resources is important when making decisions, it cannot replace knowledge of the differences in the primary outcome itself.

As comparative outcome studies can be difficult, the use of proxy measures for patient outcome has been proposed. One set of such studies takes the decision of clinicians as the outcome, while others have focused on the level of uncertainty expressed by the physician.

For far too long, decision-makers have relied on accuracy data only. Well-designed randomized studies on medical tests are possible, and their use should be encouraged. A more elaborate discussion of randomized designs for diagnostic tests can be found elsewhere (25).

MODELING APPROACHES

One other problem of randomized comparative designs is that the inclusion of a large number of patients prevents the number of strategies that can be compared. Because the end financial gain is very substantial, this is less of a problem when studying the effectiveness of pharmaceuticals; however, the need for large numbers is a challenge when looking at diagnostic tests where financial gain may be minimal.

Even if two dichotomous tests are evaluated and a dichotomous decision regarding diagnosis is required, then there are already many strategies that can be compared:

- Use test A only.
- Use B only.
- Use both A and B and rely on the combined outcome.
- Start with A and use B in test A negatives only.
- Start with A and use B in test A positives only.
- Start with B and use A in test B negatives only.
- Start with B and use A in test B positives only.

This is far too much for any randomized clinical trial. The problem grows larger quickly when more tests are considered and when tests produce quantitative (continuous) rather than black or white results.

Modeling has been proposed as an alternative approach for comparing test strategies. The researcher extracts data from the published literature on the test of interest and incorporates them into a decision analytic model, where there is virtually no limit to the number of strategies that can be compared.

Yet modeling also has its drawbacks. Modeling itself cannot eliminate any form of bias in the source data. Many decision models rely on estimates from noncomparative studies, which can be subject to all forms of selection bias and produce indirect estimates of the relative effectiveness of tests. The problem is aggravated as differences between strategies can be expected to be very small, and tiny forms of bias affect the robustness and the credibility of the results.

A different form is the use of multivariable regression models to find optimal diagnostic algorithms. Logistic regression of multiple diagnostic tests results, using the reference standard outcome as the dependent variable, is gaining popularity.

LEVELS OF EVIDENCE

In this era of evidence-based medicine, more and more decision-makers rely on the explicit, judicious, and conscientious use of the best available evidence when making decision about medical tests. To ease the construction of recommendations on diagnostic tests, a number of groups have constructed summary "levels of evidence." The most influential one can be found on the internet, at the site of the Oxford NHS R&D Centre for Evidence-Based Medicine[1] (Table 1).

These levels of evidence incorporate a number of the issues discussed in this chapter. In addition, they look at the amount of the available evidence. Systematic reviews summarizing the data from multiple studies rank higher than single studies, especially if the results from the studies in the review show a considerable amount of heterogeneity (*see* chapter 8).

Some caution is appropriate when considering the use of these levels of evidence:

- They do not look at the size of diagnostic accuracy, just at the study type and the amount of studies. In this, they do not differ from the levels of evidence for other problems.

1. Generated by discussions between Bob Phillips, Chris Ball, Dave Sackett, Brian Haynes, Sharon Straus, Finlay McAlister, and others.

Table 1
Levels of evidence for diagnostic tests

Grade of recommendation	Level of evidence	Evidence
A	1a	Systematic review (with homogeneity[a]) of prospective cohort studies; clinical decision rule[b] with 1b studies from different clinical centers
	1b	Prospective cohort study[c] with good reference standards[d] or followup; clinical decision rule tested within one clinical center
	1c	Absolute SpPins and SnNouts[e]
B	2a	Systematic review (with homogeneity[a]) of level >2 diagnostic studies
	2b	Exploratory[c] cohort study with good reference standards (1); Clinical decision rule after derivation, or validated only on split-sample or databases
	3a	Systematic review (with homogeneity[a]) of 3b and better studies
	3b	Nonconsecutive study; or without consistently applied reference standards
C	4	Case-control study, poor or nonindependent reference standard
D	5	Expert opinion without explicit critical appraisal, or based on physiology, bench research, or "first principles"

[a]A homogeneous systematic review is free of worrisome variability (heterogeneity) in the directions and degrees of results between individual studies.

[b]Clinical decision rule: an algorithm or scoring system which leads to a prognostic estimation or a diagnostic category.

[c]Validating studies test the quality of a specific diagnostic test, based on prior evidence. An exploratory study collects information and trawls the data (e.g., using a regression analysis) to find which factors are "significant."

[d]Good reference standards are independent of the test and applied blindly or objectively to all patients. Poor reference standards are haphazardly applied but are still independent of the test. Use of a nonindependent reference standard (where the test is included in the reference, or where the testing affects the reference) implies a level 4 study.

[e]An "Absolute SpPin" is a diagnostic finding whose specificity is so high that a positive result rules in the diagnosis. An "Absolute SnNout" is a diagnostic finding whose sensitivity is so high that a negative result rules out the diagnosis.

From Oxford Centre for Evidence-Based Medicine (http://www.cebm.net)

- They do not look at comparative designs, in contrast with the levels of evidence for therapy.
- They do not consider patient outcome in any form.
- They do not incorporate the consistency between accuracy data and other evidence on tests.

SUMMARY

A two-by-two table is not sufficient to obtain a test's sensitivity and specificity. The design of a diagnostic accuracy study is critically important, as design flaws can produce biased estimates. Various sources of bias in diagnostic studies have been identified. Furthermore, test properties are not fixed characteristics of a test. Even unbiased estimates will vary beyond chance, depending on the circumstances.

The evidence to support the introduction and use of medical tests should not be limited to the traditional test characteristics. Instead the downstream consequences of using test information should be explored. That should come from comparative studies, in which test results are used to guide further decisions in one group of patients, and the results of other tests—or no tests at all—in a second group, after which outcomes and the use of resources are compared.

Many today—including patients, physicians, payers, and other professionals—expect decisions to be based on strong evidence, coming from valid high-quality research. Specifying the type of evidence required and judging whether any form of research has been able to deliver that evidence requires a good understanding of the decision to be made, the available options and alternatives, the corresponding data needs, as well as a proper appreciation of the methodology for conducting and analyzing diagnostic studies. As the need for solid evidence grows, further development of this methodology can be expected in the years to come.

EXERCISES

1. Search the literature for a paper on a favorite test. Use the STARD checklist to see whether relevant items are included. Discuss for each of the STARD items whether or not there is potential for bias or lack of applicability.
2. Examine the paper—and other sources—for signs or evidence on variability in diagnostic accuracy between relevant subgroups for this test.
3. Draw the basic randomized design elements for a randomized comparative study on a favorite test, aimed at documenting changes in patient outcome from using the test. Include the comparator strategy in the design, as well as the relevant outcome measure(s). Discuss whether or not such a design is ethically or practically feasible, and discuss possible alternative designs.

4. Search the literature using PubMed to see whether any comparative studies have been performed on this test. Discuss the potential explanations for the lack of studies.

REFERENCES

1. Begg CB. Biases in the assessment of diagnostic tests. Statistics in medicine 1987;6:411–23.
2. Lijmer JG, Mol BW, Heisterkamp S, Bonsel GJ, Prins MH, Van der Meulen JH, et al. Empirical evidence of design-related bias in studies of diagnostic tests. J Am Med Assoc. 1999;282:1061–6.
3. Mower WR. Evaluating bias and variability in diagnostic test reports. Ann Emerg Med 1999;33:85–91.
4. Ransohoff DF, Feinstein AR. Problems of spectrum and bias in evaluating the efficacy of diagnostic tests. N Engl J Med 1978;299:926–30.
5. Sackett DL, Haynes RB. The architecture of diagnostic research. BMJ 2002;324:539–41.
6. Guyatt GH, Tugwell PX, Feeny DH, Haynes RB, Drummond M. A framework for clinical evaluation of diagnostic technologies. Can Med Assoc J 1986;134:587–94.
7. Smith TP. Pulmonary embolism: what's wrong with this diagnosis? AJR Am J Roentgenol 2000;174:1489–97.
8. Egermayer P. Follow-up for death or recurrence is not a reliable way of assessing the accuracy of diagnostic tests for thromboembolic disease. Chest 1997;111:1410–3.
9. Baker SG. Evaluating multiple diagnostic tests with partial verification. Biometrics 1995;51:330–7.
10. Begg CB, Greenes RA. Assessment of diagnostic tests when disease verification is subject to selection bias. Biometrics 1983;39:207–15.
11. Knottnerus JA. The effects of disease verification and referral on the relationship between symptoms and diseases. Med Dec Making 1987;7:139–48.
12. Revesz G, Kundel HL, Bonitatibus M. The effect of verification on the assessment of imaging techniques. Invest Radiol 1983;18:194–8.
13. Moons KG, Grobbee DE. When should we remain blind and when should our eyes remain open in diagnostic studies? J Clin Epidemiol 2002;55:633–6.
14. Egglin TK, Feinstein AR. Context bias. A problem in diagnostic radiology. JAMA 1996;276:1752–5.
15. Habbema JDF ER, Krijnen P, Knottnerus JA. Analysis of data on the accuracy of diagnostic tests. In: Knottnerus JA, ed. The evidence base of clinial diagnosis. London: BMJ Books, 2002.
16. Irwig L, Bossuyt P, Glasziou P, Gatsonis C, Lijmer J. Designing studies to ensure that estimates of test accuracy are transferable. BMJ 2002;324:669–71.
17. Scouller K, Conigrave KM, Macaskill P, Irwig L, Whitfield JB. Should we use carbohydrate-deficient transferrin instead of gamma-glutamyltransferase for detecting problem drinkers? A systematic review and metaanalysis. Clin Chem 2000;46:1894–902.
18. Moher D, Schulz KF, Altman DG. The CONSORT statement: revised

recommendations for improving the quality of reports of parallel-group randomized trials. Ann Intern Med 2001;134:657–62.

19. Bossuyt PM, Reitsma JB, Bruns DE, Gatsonis CA, Glasziou PP, Irwig LM, et al. Towards complete and accurate reporting of studies of diagnostic accuracy: The STARD Initiative. *Radiology* 2003;226:24–8.

20. Bossuyt PM, Reitsma JB, Bruns DE, Gatsonis CA, Glasziou PP, Irwig LM, et al. The STARD statement for reporting studies of diagnostic accuracy: explanation and elaboration. Clin Chem 2003;49:7–18.

21. Knottnerus J, Dinant G-J, van Schayk O. The diagnostic before-after study to assess clinical impact. In: Knottnerus J, Ed. The Evidence Base of Clinical Diagnosis. London: BMJ Books, 2002.

22. Guyatt GH, Tugwell PX, Feeny DH, Drummond MF, Haynes RB. The role of before-after studies of therapeutic impact in the evaluation of diagnostic technologies. J Chronic Dis 1986;39:295–304.

23. Hunink MG, Krestin GP. Study design for concurrent development, assessment, and implementation of new diagnostic imaging technology. Radiology 2002;222:604–14.

24. Bossuyt PM, Lijmer JG, Mol BW. Randomised comparisons of medical tests: sometimes invalid, not always efficient. Lancet 2000;356:1844–7.

25. Lijmer JG, Bossuyt PM. Diagnostic testing and prognosis: the randomized controlled trial in diagnostic research. In: Knottnerus JA, ed. The evidence base of clinical diagnosis. London: BMJ Books, 2002.

6

Searching the Literature and Relevant Databases

Atle Klovning and Sverre Sandberg

Just why are searches needed? Practicing evidence-based laboratory medicine requires integration of clinical skills and experience with current best evidence, which then has to be combined with patient values and choices. The challenge for modern laboratory medicine is to find and apply the best evidence. Electronic access to databases and journals makes information easily retrievable and solves the issue of finding current best evidence. On the other hand, searches may yield too much data and result in information overload. A structured approach is needed to filtering valid and reliable information from data that are not useful.

For searches to be useful, they must be correctly designed and executed. Much work has been put into the process of systematically reviewing literature for therapeutic interventions and compiling valid and rigorous information sources for busy clinicians, resulting in resources such as the Cochrane Library (CL), Clinical Evidence (CE), and the American College of Physicians Journal Club (ACPJC, formerly known as Best Evidence). Much less effort has been put into systematizing the diagnostics literature. If a search is incorrectly performed, relevant information may be missed, or huge masses of irrelevant material might be retrieved.

This chapter provides a practical introduction to searching the literature, points out where to search for diagnostic literature, and explains how to perform searches in different databases. The focus is on electronically accessible resources, since these are widely accessible through Internet connections. A search strategy is developed systematically and applied to a comprehensive search for the most up-to-date literature on diagnostic tests. And finally, validations of these search strategies are detailed.

DESIGNING THE SEARCH

The design of a search requires knowledge of appropriate search terms and where to find them. In addition, some tips for searching and browsing are provided.

Finding Search Terms

Generally, a sensitive search would require combining keywords like medical subject headings (MeSH terms) with free text words. Most databases and search engines use similar methods for conducting searches. Medline and the Cochrane Library use index terms like MeSH and also allow the use of free terms or text words and field delimiters like date, age, and publication type. One excellent source for information on how to perform searches is found in the Cochrane Library's help file. Free access to a similar source is found in the PubMed help file. Readers should look up the specific help files of the systems they use. Some example MeSH search terms are listed in the accompanying boxes.

General Tips for Searching and Browsing

To start with, enter a term in a search window, and then click on the button labeled "Search." In combined databases, multiple databases and resources

---

MeSH Terms

SENSITIVITY-AND-SPECIFICITY
RADIOLOGY-DIAGNOSTIC-X-RAY see RADIOGRAPHY
ROUTINE-DIAGNOSTIC-TESTS see DIAGNOSTIC-TESTS-ROUTINE
IMAGING-DIAGNOSTIC see DIAGNOSTIC-IMAGING
DIAGNOSTIC-EQUIPMENT
DIAGNOSTIC-ERRORS
DIAGNOSTIC-IMAGING
REAGENT-KITS-DIAGNOSTIC

X-RAY-DIAGNOSTIC see RADIOGRAPHY
DIAGNOSTIC-REAGENT-KITS see REAGENT-KITS-DIAGNOSTIC
MASS-SCREENING
DIAGNOSTIC-SERVICES
DIAGNOSTIC-TECHNIQUES-AND-PROCEDURES
DIAGNOSTIC-TECHNIQUES-CARDIOVASCULAR
DIAGNOSTIC-TECHNIQUES-DIGESTIVE-SYSTEM
DIAGNOSTIC-TECHNIQUES-ENDOCRINE
DIAGNOSTIC-TECHNIQUES-NEUROLOGICAL
DIAGNOSTIC-TECHNIQUES-OBSTETRICAL-AND-GYNECOLOGICAL
DIAGNOSTIC-TECHNIQUES-OPHTHALMOLOGICAL
DIAGNOSTIC-TECHNIQUES-OTOLOGICAL
DIAGNOSTIC-TECHNIQUES-RADIOISOTOPE
DIAGNOSTIC-TECHNIQUES-RESPIRATORY-SYSTEM
DIAGNOSTIC-TECHNIQUES-SURGICAL
DIAGNOSTIC-TECHNIQUES-UROLOGICAL
LABORATORY-TECHNIQUES-AND-SCREENING
DIAGNOSTIC-TESTS-ROUTINE
REFERENCE-VALUE

MeSH Subheadings

http://www.ncbi.nlm.nih.gov:80/entrez/query/static/help/pmhelp.html#subheadingslist

Analogs and Derivatives	AA	Legislation and Jurisprudence	LJ
Abnormalities	AB	Manpower	MA
Administration and Dosage	AD	Metabolism	ME
Adverse Effects	AE	Microbiology	MI
Agonists	AG	Mortality	MO
Anatomy and Histology	AH	Methods	MT
Antagonists and Inhibitors	AI	Nursing	NU
Analysis	AN	Organization and Administration	OG
Biosynthesis	BI	Pathology	PA
Blood	BL	Prevention and Control	PC
Blood Supply	BS	Pharmacology	PD
Cerebrospinal Fluid	CF	Physiology	PH
Chemistry	CH	Pharmacokinetics	PK
Chemically Induced	CI	Poisoning	PO
Classification	CL	Physiopathology	PP
Congenital	CN	Parasitology	PS
Complications	CO	Psychology	PX
Chemical Synthesis	CS	Pathogenicity	PY
Contraindications	CT	Radiography	RA
Cytology	CY	Radiation Effects	RE
Drug Effects	DE	Rehabilitation	RH
Deficiency	DF	Radionuclide Imaging	RI
Diet Therapy	DH	Radiotherapy	RT
Diagnosis	DI	Secondary	SC
Drug Therapy	DT	Supply and Distribution	SD
Diagnostic Use	DU	Secretion	SE
Economics	EC	Statistics and Numerical Data	SN
Education	ED	Standards	ST
Ethnology	EH	Surgery	SU
Embryology	EM	Trends	TD
Enzymology	EN	Therapy	TH
Epidemiology	EP	Transmission	TM
Ethics	ES	Toxicity	TO
Etiology	ET	Transplantation	TR
Growth and Development	GD	Therapeutic Use	TU
Genetics	GE	Ultrastructure	UL
History	HI	Urine	UR
Immunology	IM	Ultrasonography	US
Injuries	IN	Utilization	UT
Isolation and Purification	IP	Veterinary	VE
Innervation	IR	Virology	VI
Instrumentation	IS		

may be searched simultaneously. The number of documents meeting the search criterion or criteria is called hits, and the total number of documents found will usually be displayed. The documents retrieved may then be viewed either by clicking on URLs (links) or by downloading documents as PDFs (portable document formats that retain all formatting and typesetting). The free, downloadable Adobe Acrobat Reader may be used to open PDFs, and usually all necessary information regarding this is given at the different sites. If no documents are found, many databases offer tips on improving searches. The subscription-based Knowledge Finder Medline at www.kfinder.com lists the hits according to "relevance." This listing can be a big help. Other Medline interfaces just list references chronologically which may be a major disadvantage due to the large number of abstracts that frequently result from the search; the large quantity makes extracting relevant, high-quality studies difficult and tedious.

Using Medical Subject Headings (MeSH)

Medline citations and Cochrane Reviews now include MeSH terms assigned by librarians at the National Library of Medicine (NLM) in the United States. Searching the databases using medical subject headings involves three steps.

Use a thesaurus function to find appropriate search words.
Select terms from the MeSH trees.
Search on the chosen term.

"Single-term" searches explore the database only for one term, while "exploded-term" searches explore all of the children of this term and in all trees. For example, searching "anemia" gives:

MeSH trees

Hemic and Lymphatic Diseases [C15]
 Hematologic Diseases [C15.378]
  Anemia [C15.378.071]
   Anemia, Hypochromic [C15.378.071.196]
   Anemia, Iron-Deficiency [C15.378.071.196.300]

Nutritional and Metabolic Diseases [C18]
 Metabolic Diseases [C18.452]
  Iron Metabolism Disorders [C18.452.565]
   Anemia, Iron-Deficiency [C18.452.565.100]
   Iron Overload [C18.452.565.500]

Non-MeSH Searches

Some terms in the MeSH index are labeled "(Non MeSH)" and start with an asterisk (*). These terms are used by indexers to group headings in the MeSH tree structures. Because they are not true index terms, they should not be used in searches.

Search History

Following each search, the search number and search term will be shown under a search history. Searches may be stored in many ways locally on one's own computer (for example, when searching PubMed with the reference manager program EndNote). Also, when searching PubMed directly, one can sign up for a "cubby save" in order to retain the search for future use. Clicking on a saved search term will directly repeat the search. Previously performed searches can be combined by entering the search numbers with combining words. The display will then show the results for the combined search; for example:

#1 cobalamin
#2 homocysteine
#3 #1 AND #2

Restricting Searches

One can restrict searches in different ways, for example, by date or publication type. As an example, in some search languages, this is done as cobalamin AND review: PT to search for a certain publication type. PT is an example of a field delimiter. Other delimiters are age categories, gender, and language.

Only Items with Abstracts

Retrieval may be limited to only citations that contain an abstract by delimiters for abstracts only, but bear in mind that citations to articles published prior to 1975 do not include abstracts.

Publication Types

All citations in PubMed are for journal articles. However, retrieval may be limited based on the type of material that the article represents (e.g., clinical trials or review articles). The "Publication Types" pull-down menu in PubMed contains a list of frequently searched publication types (i.e., clinical trial, editorial, letter, meta-analysis, practice guideline, randomized controlled trial, and review). If no selection is made, PubMed will not restrict the search to any particular publication type.

If the Publication Types pull-down menu is used to select a search field, then the retrieval will be limited to Medline citations. Thus, Pre-Medline "in process" and "supplied by publisher" citations will be excluded because they have not yet completed the indexing process and will therefore not include a publication type.

Age as Delimiter

To select a specific age group for human studies, click on the "Ages" pull-down menu and select from one of the age groups listed (Table 1). If no selection is made, PubMed will not limit retrieval by age groups.

Refining Your Search

There are several ways to make a search more specific, retrieving less irrelevant material. To do this when conducting a search using more than one word, several rules apply. The first is that all text must be searched in the default setting (e.g., titles, abstracts, authors' names, citations, and keywords). Remember that case may be ignored, stop words are ignored, all numbers are ignored, and punctuation at the beginning and end of words is ignored.

Some other things to remember:

Wildcards: Wildcards may be asterisks (*), dollar signs ($), or question marks (?), depending on the database being used. The asterisk symbol acts as a wildcard that matches all words that begin with the string of

Table 1
Medline age categories

Medline term	How it restricts the search
All infant	Birth–23 months
All child	0–18 years
All adult	19+ years
Newborn	Birth–1 month
Infant	1–23 months
Preschool child	2–5 years
Child	6–12 years
Adolescent	13–18 years
Adult	19–44 years
Middle aged	45–64 years
Middle aged + aged	45+ years
Aged	65+ years
80 and over	80+ years

characters before the asterisk. For example, cobal* searches both cobalamin and cobalt.

Apostrophes (phrase searching): Other search engines want the search words enclosed with apostrophes. The search is "read" from left to right unless brackets are used to group words. Each word is considered individually by default when searching. Just searching iron deficiency would give iron AND deficiency. Using quotation marks/apostrophes lets the user search iron deficiency if the terms are enclosed like this: "iron deficiency" as the search term. This is especially important in Internet search engines. Also, when a phrase is enclosed in double quotes, PubMed will not perform automatic term mapping. Normally, unqualified terms that are entered in the query box are matched (in this order) first against a MeSH Translation Table. If no MeSH term is found, the search is mapped against a Journals Translation Table, or finally an Author Index

Retrieving all records: An asterisk entered on its own will retrieve all records in the database. To retrieve all records published in 1995, for example, enter * as a search term, and limit the date range to 1995. Alternatively, just click "Search" with nothing entered in the search window.

Combining Searches

Search terms can be combined using the Boolean words: AND, OR, NOT, NEAR, and NEXT. It must be noted that terms may differ in other searching systems. Often the combining terms have to be written in capital letters and care also must be taken when using brackets.

AND: By default, records are selected as if they were joined by AND. This retrieves records containing the search terms anywhere in the text of the record (e.g., iron deficiency equals iron AND deficiency).

OR: Enter "OR" between words to select records containing any of the word(s) in the search string. For example, homocysteine OR cobalamin will retrieve all records containing homocysteine and all records containing cobalamin, whether or not these records contain both words.

NEXT or ADJ: The operator NEXT (ADJ in some systems) will link the words on either side of the word NEXT, in the order they are specified. For example,. "iron NEXT deficiency" is not the same as "deficiency NEXT iron."

NEAR: The operator NEAR works in a similar way to NEXT, searching words that are within six words of each other. For example, "iron NEAR anemia" will pick up phrases such as: "Iron deficiency in women with anemia was found to be . . .." The order of the words either side of NEAR is not important. For example, "deficiency NEAR anemia" will pick up the same documents as "anemia NEAR deficiency."

Great care has to be taken if OR, AND, or NOT is used in the same search as NEAR or NEXT; some impossible combinations may arise.

RESOURCES FOR SEARCHES ON DIAGNOSTIC TESTS

Although there are numerous databases that can be searched, it is critically important to bear in mind that relevant evidence may not be electronically accessible. Links can change and new databases may appear; updated information can be found at http://www.cmwr.org/ebm/. Some databases are free and some are commercial; also, some are single databases, while others are combined databases. When conducting systematic reviews, it is necessary to consult colleagues or field experts to get information on potentially useful databases. Furthermore, unpublished studies may be located by examining bibliographies of identified articles and literature from governmental institutions, by personal contact with collaborators, or more systematically through postal surveys to academic departments and researchers worldwide that are active or interested in the field (1).

The following resources are ranked according to the methodologic quality of information obtainable in each. The highest methodologic quality is designated level 1, and the lowest quality is listed as level 7. All levels may provide useful information and should be searched when conducting systematic reviews. The busy laboratorian, however, would probably find aggregated information at level 1 or 2 most useful.

1. The Cochrane Library

URL: http://www.cochrane.org
The Cochrane Library contains seven databases; the DARE database is the most relevant for diagnostic tests:

- The Cochrane Database of Systematic Reviews (CDSR)
- The Database of Abstracts of Reviews of Effectiveness (DARE)
- The NHS Economic Evaluation Database
- The Cochrane Database of Methodology Reviews
- Health Technology Assessment Database
- The Cochrane Central Register of Controlled Trials (CENTRAL)
- The Cochrane Methodology Register (formerly called the Review Methodology Database)

The Cochrane Library has some CDSRs on tests, but more are found in DARE, and the economic evaluation databases are often useful.

2. Secondary Journals and Databases

A number of useful resources are available. Here are some of the more important ones.

Clinical Evidence
URL: www.clinicalevidence.com
So far, all effort has been put into summarizing information from therapeutic trials. The rigorous methods applied make this a primary source. In the future, efforts will be made to include information on diagnostic procedures.

ACP Journal Club (formerly Best Evidence)
URL: www.acpjc.org
ACP Journal Club cites and critically appraises well-performed and valid studies and also has a focus on diagnostic studies.

Bandolier
URL: www.jr2.ox.ac.uk/bandolier/
This secondary journal provides evidence-based summaries and comments, even on diagnostic issues.

TRIP Database
URL: www.tripdatabase.com
This database provides evidence-based summaries with comments, also on diagnostic issues.

3. Medline Searches

Searches using Medline are convenient. The following provides some specific information to make its use more meaningful.

PubMed
URL: www.pubmed.com
PubMed is free and allows use of validated search filters for selecting papers on diagnosis, etiology, prognosis, and therapy. Search filters were constructed by Haynes et al. (2) and have been validated (3–5).

MeSH subheadings [sh] are used with MeSH terms [mh] to help describe more completely a particular aspect of a subject. For example, the drug therapy for asthma is displayed as asthma/drug therapy. Another example: ANEMIA-IRON-DEFICIENCY [mh] AND DIAGNOSIS [sh]. MeSH subheadings automatically include the more specific subheading terms under the term in a search. To turn off this automatic feature in PubMed, use the search syntax [sh: noexp], e.g., diagnosis [sh: noexp]. It is also possible to enter the Medline two-letter MeSH subheading abbreviations shown in the provided box, rather than spelling out the subheading, e.g., di [sh] = diagnosis [sh].

Clinical Queries

URL: http://www.ncbi.nlm.nih.gov:80/entrez/query/static/clinical.html
PubMed's evidence-based search filters were developed by Haynes and co-workers (2, 3); with these, Medline can be searched with two filters. One filter is sensitive and provides many papers, of which many may not be relevant. The other filter is constructed for high specificity and yields fewer papers, possibly missing some that are relevant. These filters have been validated (1, 4–6). The PubMed clinical queries interface provides the necessary filters by means of a simple click on a button. Searches are a balance; they may be sensitive, finding many studies including a number of irrelevant ones, or specific, finding fewer studies but missing some that may be relevant.

OVID

URL: http://www.ovid.com/index.cfm
OVID is a commercial database with access to evidence-based resource material (EBRM). It gives access to EMBASE, one of the major databases needed for performing searches when doing systematic reviews.

Medline at NLM

URL: http://www.nlm.nih.gov/
The Medline database may be searched with different interfaces, and it now includes Pre-Medline. If a search is needed for articles published in the last couple of weeks, try searching Pre-Medline. Pre-Medline citations are not indexed, so text word searches are used to retrieve them. Pre-Medline is the National Library of Medicine's in-process database for Medline. It provides basic citation information and abstracts before the citation is indexed with NLM's MeSH heading and added to Medline. Records will appear with the tag "MEDLINE record in process" until they are available in full form in the Medline database. It is a vital resource for medical researchers who need up-to-the-minute information, and it is updated daily as part of the OVID Biomed Service. Pre-Medline is also available as part of the NLM PubMed service to all users without registration. Once subject headings and other relevant data are added, the article's complete record is incorporated into the full Medline database and removed from Pre-Medline. Records supplied by the publisher are added daily to Pre-Medline but have not yet gone through NLM's quality control process. As with Medline, the scope of Pre-Medline is biomedical. It provides coverage of all articles that are indexed in Medline. Pre-Medline is basically a processing database for Medline and contains 25,000–100,000 records at any time.

Knowledge Finder Medline (subscription-based)
URL: http://www.kfinder.com
This version of Medline allows the user to enter well-formulated English language questions into the search field. The search is then converted into MeSH terms, and by means of fuzzy logic, a list of Medline papers is retrieved. The topmost are ranked as the most relevant papers, and the results of the search are shown graphically, depicted by a blue bar. For a quick Medline search, this option is ideal. When searching for diagnostic studies, it is helpful to include "predictive value" in the sentence.

4. Primary Journals (Free versus Paid Access)

The site for free online medical journals is found at the URL: www.freemedicaljournals.com. Access to many journals has been prepaid at many university locations.

e-BMJ
URL: http://www.bmj.com
The *British Medical Journal* prepared the groundwork for free Internet access to its journal. Many collaborating journals use the same web-platform, allowing cross-searching into a vast number of journals via BMJ.

Clinical Chemistry
URL: http://www.clinchem.org/
This journal is of vital importance and has a section on evidence-based laboratory medicine and test utilization. There is also an option for multiple-journal search.

5. Guidelines

There are many sources for guidelines for therapeutic interventions but not as many for diagnostic strategies. However, some health technology assessment documents on screening tests take the form of guidelines. Some useful sites are:

- Agency for Healthcare Research and Quality http://www.ahcpr.gov/clinic/
- National Guideline Clearinghouse www.guideline.gov
- Primary Care Internet Guide http://www.uib.no/isf/guide/misc.htm

6. Internet Search Engines

There are numerous search engines that vary in the material that they cover. The Internet has grown so quickly and is so large that discerning between high- and low-quality information is not an easy task. Some potentially useful examples of search engines and their addresses are:

- Google **www.google.com**
- AltaVista **www.AltaVista.com**
- FAST **www.alltheweb.com**
- Yahoo **www.yahoo.com**

7. Academic Discussion Groups

At http://www.jiscmail.ac.uk/, there are thousands of academic e-mail lists; an especially important one is the evidence-based-health discussion list. See http://www.cmwr.org/ebm/ for instructions on how to join this or other lists. Having performed the previous steps when searching for evidence, one could ask members of the group for references or discussion on a specific topic.

Examples

The first challenge is to know where to search for diagnostic tests; the second challenge is how to perform optimal searches in order to find valid, useful, and up-to-date resources. The process starts with formulating a question, then developing a search strategy, deciding which databases to search, and then finally conducting the search.

Example: What is the usefulness of Helicobacter pylori tests in primary healthcare?

The Cochrane Library
Find the terms in the Thesaurus. They are helicobacter-pylori and primary-health-care; combine them with "AND."
Enter: Helicobacter, select exploded. The following will be returned:

Search term: HELICOBACTER-PYLORI*:ME [No restrictions]

What you get in the Cochrane Library search is shown in the accompanying box.

If this is combined with primary-health-care, six randomized controlled trials are retrieved in the CENTRAL database, and one economic evaluation.

Knowledge Finder Medline
What is the usefulness of *Helicobacter pylori* tests in primary healthcare?
By means of concept mapping and fuzzy logic, the first hits listed are "presumed" to be the most relevant and useful ones. Cross out the ones of inter-

Results from The Cochrane Library

The Cochrane Database of Systematic Reviews (CDSR)
Complete reviews   0 [1596]
Protocols   0 [1200]

Database of Abstracts of Reviews of Effectiveness (DARE)
Abstracts of quality assessed systematic reviews   4 [3075]
Other reviews: bibliographic details only   1 [800]

The Cochrane Central Register of Controlled Trials (CENTRAL)
References   42 [353809]

The Cochrane Database of Methodology Reviews
Complete reviews   0 [8]
Protocols   0 [7]

The Cochrane Methodology Register
References   0 [4388]

About the Cochrane Collaboration
The Cochrane Collaboration   0 [1]

Collaborative Review Groups — CRGs   0 [50]
Fields   0 [9]
Methods Groups   0 [10]
Networks   0 [1]
Centres   0 [13]

Health Technology Assessment Database (HTA)
Abstracts by INAHTA and other healthcare technology agencies   0 [2870]
NHS Economic Evaluation Database (NHS EED)
Critically appraised economic evaluations   20 [4078]
Other economic studies: bibliographic details   4 [6878]

est, download them to a reference-managing program, or e-mail the list as shown in Figure 1.

PubMed Clinical Queries

Searching with the term "Helicobacter pylori" AND "Primary Health Care" using the specificity filter for diagnosis together with the systematic review filter turns the search into: (Primary-health-care and helicobacter-pylori) AND (sensitivity and specificity [MeSH] OR (predictive [WORD] AND value* [WORD])), yielding 13 highly relevant studies when using the specificity filter. When the specificity filter is replaced by the sensitivity filter, the search is converted into: (Primary-health-care and helicobacter-pylori) AND (sensitivity and specificity [MeSH] OR sensitiv-

---

From: atle.klovning@isf.uib.no
Date: Sunday March 23, 2003 15:14:14
To: atle.klovning@isf.uib.no
Topic: hpyl
Answer to: atle.klovning@isf.uib.no

Forwarded to you from Aries Systems Corporation <KWEB-SERVER> at the request of
< atle.klovning@isf.uib.no >

08 SERIAL TI : Aliment Pharmacol Ther 2001 Aug;15(8):1205-10
15 ARTICLE AU : Weijnen CF; De Wit NJ; Numans ME; Kuipers EJ; Hoes AW; Verheij TJ
16 ARTICLE TI : Helicobacter pylori testing in the primary care setting: which diagnostic test should be used?

08 SERIAL TI : Helicobacter 1998 Sep;3(3):179-83
15 ARTICLE AU : Hackelsberger A; Schultze V; Peitz U; Gunther T; Nilius M; Diete U; Schumacher M; Roessner A; Malfertheiner P
16 ARTICLE TI : Performance of a rapid whole blood test for Helicobacter pylori in primary care: a German multicenter study.

08 SERIAL TI : BMJ 1998 May 2;316(7141):1389
15 ARTICLE AU : Churchill RD; Hill PG; Holmes GK
16 ARTICLE TI : Management of dyspepsia in primary care. Breath test is better than near patient blood tests.

08 SERIAL TI : Br J Gen Pract 2000 Jan;50(450):13-6
15 ARTICLE AU : Quartero AO; Numans ME; de Melker RA; de Wit NJ
16 ARTICLE TI : In-practice evaluation of whole-blood Helicobacter pylori test: its usefulness in detecting peptic ulcer disease.

08 SERIAL TI : Med Decis Making 2003 Jan-Feb;23(1):21-30
15 ARTICLE AU : Delaney BC; Holder RL; Allan TF; Kenkre JE; Hobbs FD
16 ARTICLE TI : A comparison of Bayesian and maximum likelihood methods to determine the performance of a point of care test for Helicobacter pylori in the office setting [In Process Citation]

Figure 1 One example of results from Knowledge Finder Medline downloaded to e-mail. PubMed (free access) also provides the same e-mail option.

ity [WORD] OR (diagnosis [SH] OR diagnostic use [SH] OR specificity [WORD])). This search will return 43 studies.

ONGOING EFFORTS

Since the early days of computerized access to Medline, many series of papers have been published by different research groups, including the productive group at McMaster University in Canada. These efforts started with "How to keep up with the literature" (7–12) in 1985, then focused on clinical use of the Medline database (13–20), and evolving into the Evidence-Based Medicine Working Group (EBMWG). The EBMWG authored the *Journal of the American Medical Association's* series of Users' Guides to diagnostic tests (21, 22) and how to use electronic resources (23) (*see also* http://www.usersguides.org/). Eventually this effort led to the Rational Clinical Examination series in the *Journal of the American Medical Association*, validating the use of different kinds of tests for multiple clinical entities.

The Cochrane Collaboration

In the process of performing systematic reviews of diagnostic tests, the Cochrane Working Group on Systematic Reviews of Screening and Diagnostic Tests was registered with the Cochrane Collaboration in October 1995. This group has prepared a document on recommended methods for performing systematic reviews of diagnostic tests, which is available on the Internet (24).

Database of Abstracts of Review of Effectiveness (DARE)

The Cochrane Collaboration has mainly focused on performing systematic reviews of therapeutic interventions, and therefore the Cochrane Database of Systematic Reviews (CDSR) is of little use concerning diagnostic tests. On the other hand, the DARE database in the Cochrane Library is a very useful resource. The Centre for Reviews and Dissemination in York (United Kingdom) has agreed to include assessments of systematic reviews of diagnostic tests in the Database of Abstracts of Review of Effectiveness (DARE). One of the useful reviews to be found here is a systematic review of near-patient testing in primary care (1), where a wide collection of sources have been searched, and the searches have been validated. For readers undertaking systematic reviews, it is a very useful example.

The Bayes Library of Diagnostic Studies and Reviews

The group preparing the Bayes Library of Diagnostic Studies and Reviews (6) will be coordinating its efforts with the team behind Clinical Evidence, the Committee on Evidence-Based Laboratory Medicine in the International Federation for Clinical Chemistry (IFCC), and the Cochrane Collaboration. Two databases will be termed the Bayes Database of Diagnostic Reviews (BDDR) and the Bayes Diagnostic Studies Register (BDSR).

Criteria for Proper Search Strategies

The ideal is to perform searches that yield high sensitivity (finding as many relevant articles as possible), and high specificity (keeping the number of irrelevant papers as low as possible). For any search, there is a trade-off between sensitivity and specificity. When performing a systematic review, high sensitivity is required, whereas a busy laboratorian addressing a certain problem may want fewer but highly relevant articles (e.g., systematic reviews) and would then desire high specificity. In the Cochrane Library, some authors of systematic reviews have used suboptimal search strategies and resources; some have even restricted searches to English language only Medline citations. A proper search strategy for a systematic review must cover all relevant databases and needs to document and validate search strategies (*see* chapter 8). Preferably, the search strategy should be validated against hand searching as the gold standard. As mentioned earlier, other important sources are unpublished material, "grey" literature produced by manufacturers, and the valuable insight of colleagues and field experts. Internet search engines and specific content databases pose other quality-of-information challenges. Finally, hand searching references from papers retrieved from databases needs to be done when doing systematic reviews, and this has been validated (25).

VALIDATION OF SEARCH STRATEGIES

As stated earlier, a sensitive search retrieves a large number of studies, where a large proportion may be irrelevant; on the other hand, a search with high specificity retrieves fewer papers but may overlook some that could be relevant. As a central part of the evidence-based medicine process, Haynes et al. (13) evaluated Medline searching systems in 1985 and studied the importance of online access for clinical use (16). When Medline access by computer became easily accessible and free of charge, there was a shift from librarian-conducted searches to end-user searches. McKibbon et al. (26) found the quality of searches was better when performed by librarians, compared to when end-users perform searches themselves. Several routes exist to Medline, with both free and commercial vendors, like OVID, which also provides access to evidence-based resources and full-text journals that are not available for free on the Internet. With end-users using the Internet for solving clinical problems, there was a need to develop optimal search strategies. Wilczynski in Haynes' group worked on developing methodologic search filters (2, 3) and also studied the effect of introducing structured abstracts, the use of pre-explosions, and the use of subheadings (27, 28). This effort has lead to the development of rigorous search strategies for use in conducting systematic reviews of diagnostic tests. Recent papers have further validated Haynes' search filters (4, 5).

Retrieval Characteristics of Methodologic Text Words and MeSH Terms

Haynes' group at McMaster University published a paper in 1993 on the retrieval characteristics of *methodologic text words*, that is, text word (tw) combinations that identify methodological types of papers, and *Medical Subject Headings* (MeSH terms) in Medline for identifying methodologically sound studies on the etiology, prognosis, diagnosis, and prevention and treatment of disorders in general adult medicine (3).

They compared methodologic search terms and phrases for the ability to retrieve citations in Medline with a manual hand search of the literature (the gold standard) for 10 internal and general medicine journals for the years 1986 and 1991. Sensitivity and specificity of the search strategies were calculated; the individual terms yielding the best sensitivity for 1991 by category are shown in Table 2.

The authors concluded that the performance of MeSH terms and methodologic text words varied greatly in Medline and even changed from 1986 to 1991. They found that more complex search strategies might be required to optimize retrieval of relevant materials (2, 3).

Optimal Search Strategies for Retrieving Sound Clinical Studies of the Etiology, Prognosis, Diagnosis, Prevention, or Treatment of Disorders

Haynes et al. (2) also published a paper on developing optimal search strategies for detecting clinically sound studies in Medline. To this end, an analytic survey of operating characteristics of search strategies, developed by computerized combinations of terms selected to detect studies meeting basic methodologic criteria for direct clinical use in adult general medicine, was performed. In this study, the sensitivities and specificities of 134,264 unique combinations of search terms were determined by comparison with a manual review of all articles (the gold standard) in 10 internal medicine

Table 2
Search terms yielding best sensitivity[a]

	1986	Sensitivity, %	1991	Sensitivity, %
Etiology	Risk (tw)	72	Risk (tw)	82
Prognosis	Prognosis (tw)	95	Exp cohort studies	92
Diagnosis	Sensitivity (tw)	86	Sensitivity (tw)	92
Treatment	Random (tw)	98	Clinical trial (pt)	99

[a]From Haynes and coworkers (2, 3). Text word, (tw); publication type, (pt).

and general medicine journals for 1986 and 1991. They found that less than half of the studies of the topics of interest met basic criteria for scientific soundness.

Compared with the best single terms, multiple terms increased sensitivity for sound studies by more than 30% (absolute increase), but with some loss of specificity. For 1986 citations, combinations reached peak sensitivities of 72% for etiology, 95% for prognosis, 86% for diagnosis, and 98% for therapy. When search terms were combined to maximize specificity, more than 93% specificity was achieved for all-purpose categories in both years.

Compared with individual search terms, combined terms achieved higher specificity that was maintained with modest increases in sensitivity in all categories except therapy. The authors concluded that selected combinations of indexing terms and text words could substantially enhance the retrieval of studies of important clinical topics cited in Medline (2).

Comparison of Pre-Explosions and Subheading with Methodologic Search Terms in Medline

Wilczynski et al. (29) performed a quantitative comparison of the use of pre-explosions and subheadings with methodologic search terms in Medline in 1994; in other words, they compared use of the main terms with use of all of the derivative-related terms. They compared the retrieval characteristics of subheadings with methodologic text words and MeSH terms in Medline for identifying sound clinical studies on the etiology, prognosis, diagnosis, prevention, and treatment of disorders.

For treatment and diagnosis in 1991, and treatment, diagnosis, and etiology in 1986, the use of pre-explosions yielded the highest sensitivity, with typical absolute increases exceeding 15% (29). For etiology and prognosis in 1991, and prognosis in 1986, text words or MeSH terms yielded the highest sensitivity.

Compared with searching with single methodologic text words and subject headings, the detection of sound clinical studies on the diagnosis and treatment of disorders in general adult medicine was consistently enhanced by searching with pre-explosions but at a price of decreased specificity (29).

Combining Free Text and MeSH Term Searching, without Restriction to the Primary Healthcare Setting

A study published in 1997 by van der Weijden et al. (30) identified relevant diagnostic studies in Medline, with the diagnostic value of the erythrocyte sedimentation rate (ESR) and urine dipstick as an example. The combined MeSH and free text search was more sensitive than MeSH term searching only for both the ESR and the dipstick search. With this combined search, sensitivities of 91 and 98% and positive predictive values of 10 and 68% were found for ESR and dipstick, respectively. By restricting the search with keywords describing the primary healthcare setting, the positive predictive values increased to 72 and 100% but sensitivity dropped to 10 and 7% (ESR and dipstick, respectively) compared with hand searching. Combining free text and MeSH term searches, without restriction to the healthcare setting, is a valuable strategy in systematically searching for available evidence on the value of a diagnostic test in the scope of a specific disease. The authors suggest that Medline should provide a term such as "diagnostic evaluation study" to be used in the limit field Publication Type to specify diagnostic studies, so that diagnostic studies might be more easily retrieved.

New Search Strategies Using MeSH terms and Free Text Words

Devillé et al. (4) developed an optimal search strategy for diagnostic test evaluations in family medicine journals. They found that search strategies for articles reporting on diagnostic test evaluations had been subjected to less research than those in the domain of clinical trials. These authors set out to develop an optimal search strategy for publications on diagnostic test evaluations in general that could be added to keywords describing the specific diagnostic test at issue. Nine family medicine journals were searched from 1992 through 1995 for primary publications on diagnostic test evaluation by hand searching and by a Medline search strategy published earlier. New search strategies were developed with stepwise logistic regression, using MeSH terms and free text words related to diagnosis and test evaluation as independent variables. Hand searching identified 75 primary publications on diagnostic test evaluation from a total of 2467 primary publications. The most accurate new search strategy had a sensitivity of 80% , a specificity of 97%, and a positive predictive value of 48%. This search strategy used the MeSH term "sensitivity and specificity" (exploded with the MeSH terms "predictive value" and "ROC"), and cumulatively added the text words "specificity," "false negative," "accuracy," and "screening."

To obtain a search with high sensitivity, for example, searching articles for systematic reviews, Bachmann et al. (5) suggested the following strategy:

(diagnos*; predict* and accura*) in combination with the MeSH term "SENSITIVITY AND SPECIFICITY." This search produced a sensitivity of 98%.

Loss of Sensitivity and Specificity of Methodologic MeSH Terms and Text Words in Medline

Wilczynski et al. (28) published a study on possible reasons for a loss of sensitivity and specificity of methodologic MeSH terms and text words in Medline. The authors compared the frequency of nonuse and misuse of relevant methodologic MeSH terms and text words among studies that met the basic criteria for clinical practice as determined by the manual review (the gold standard) with those that did not. All articles in 10 internal and general medicine journals for 1986 and 1991 were reviewed. Loss of sensitivity due to the nonuse of relevant methodologic terms among articles meeting basic methodologic criteria was more pronounced in the areas of diagnosis, prognosis, and etiology than treatment in 1991 and 1986. The use of relevant methodologic terms improved from 1986 to 1991 in all areas except prognosis. Loss of specificity due to the use of relevant methodologic terms among articles that did not meet basic methodologic criteria occurred most frequently in the areas of treatment and etiology. Although the appropriate use of methodologic MeSH and text words has improved from 1986 to 1991 among studies meeting basic methodologic criteria for direct clinical use, much improvement is still needed in the areas of diagnosis, prognosis, and etiology. Improvement is needed in assigning the relevant methodologic index terms to studies that meet the methods criteria, and in having the authors use the relevant methodologic text words in the title or abstract. Some improvement is also needed in not using methodologic terms when the study clearly does not meet the methods criteria.

SUMMARY

Literature represents the fundamental raw material in evidence-based medicine, and critical appraisal refines this raw material to a useful product. The strategy for finding relevant and valid evidence depends on questions and information needs. Searching for diagnostic test studies requires the use of various databases. The busy laboratorian might find prefiltered databases like the TRIP database useful, while colleagues undertaking systematic reviews of the literature on diagnostic tests need to use complex and preferably validated searches (4, 6).

REFERENCES

1. Hobbs F, Delaney B, Fitzmaurice D, Wilson S, Hyde CJ, Thorpe GH, et al. A review of near patient testing in primary care. Health Technol Assess 1997;1(5):1–231.
2. Haynes RB, Wilczynski N, McKibbon KA, Walker CJ, Sinclair JC. Developing

optimal search strategies for detecting clinically sound studies in MEDLINE. J Am Med Inform Assoc 1994;1:447–58.

3. Wilczynski NL, Walker CJ, McKibbon KA, Haynes RB. Assessment of methodologic search filters in MEDLINE. Proc Annu Symp Comput Appl Med Care 1993:601–5.

4. Devillé W, Bezemer P, Bouter L. Publications on diagnostic test evaluation in family medicine journals: an optimal search strategy. J Clin Epidemiol 2000;53:65–9.

5. Bachmann L, Coray R, Estermann P, Ter RG. Identifying Diagnostic Studies in MEDLINE: Reducing the Number Needed to Read. J Am Med Inform Assoc 2002;9:653–8.

6. Battaglia M, Bucher H, Egger M, Grossenbacher F, Minder C, Pewsner D. The Bayes Library of Diagnostic Studies and Reviews. Basel: Division of Clinical Epidemiology and Biostatistics, Institute of Social and Preventive Medicine, University of Berne and Basel Institute for Clinical Epidemiology, University of Basel, Switzerland; 2002.

7. Haynes RB, McKibbon KA, Fitzgerald D, Guyatt GH, Walker CJ, Sackett DL. How to keep up with the medical literature: VI. How to store and retrieve articles worth keeping. Ann Intern Med 1986;105:978–84.

8. Haynes RB, McKibbon KA, Fitzgerald D, Guyatt GH, Walker CJ, Sackett DL. How to keep up with the medical literature: V. Access by personal computer to the medical literature. Ann Intern Med 1986;105:810–6.

9. Haynes RB, McKibbon KA, Fitzgerald D, Guyatt GH, Walker CJ, Sackett DL. How to keep up with the medical literature: IV. Using the literature to solve clinical problems. Ann Intern Med 1986;105:636–40.

10. Haynes RB, McKibbon KA, Fitzgerald D, Guyatt GH, Walker CJ, Sackett DL. How to keep up with the medical literature: III. Expanding the number of journals you read regularly. Ann Intern Med 1986;105:474–8.

11. Haynes RB, McKibbon KA, Fitzgerald D, Guyatt GH, Walker CJ, Sackett DL. How to keep up with the medical literature: II. Deciding which journals to read regularly. Ann Intern Med 1986;105:309–12.

12. Haynes RB, McKibbon KA, Fitzgerald D, Guyatt GH, Walker CJ, Sackett DL. How to keep up with the medical literature: I. Why try to keep up and how to get started. Ann Intern Med 1986;105:149–53.

13. Haynes RB, McKibbon KA, Walker CJ, Mousseau J, Baker LM, Fitzgerald D. Computer searching of the medical literature. An evaluation of MEDLINE searching systems. Ann Intern Med 1985;103:812–6.

14. McKibbon KA, Haynes RB, Baker LM, Fleming T, Walker C. Teaching clinicians to search MEDLINE: description and evaluation of a short course. Proc Annu Conf Res Med Educ 1986;25:231–6.

15. Haynes RB, McKibbon KA, Walker CJ. Planning for the information age: a survey of microcomputer use in a faculty of health sciences. Cmaj 1987;136:1035–7.

16. Haynes RB, McKibbon KA, Walker CJ, Ryan N, Fitzgerald D, Ramsden MF. Online access to MEDLINE in clinical settings. A study of use and usefulness. Ann Intern Med 1990;112:78–84.

17. Haynes RB, McKibbon KA, Walker CJ, Ramsden MF. Rapid evolution of microcomputer use in a faculty of health sciences. Cmaj 1991;144:24–8.

18. McKibbon KA, Haynes RB, Johnston ME, Walker CJ. A study to enhance clinical end-user MEDLINE search skills: design and baseline findings. Proc Annu Symp Comput Appl Med Care 1991:73–7.
19. Walker CJ, McKibbon KA, Haynes RB, Ramsden MF. Problems encountered by clinical end users of MEDLINE and GRATEFUL MED. Bull Med Libr Assoc 1991;79:67–9.
20. Haynes RB, Johnston ME, McKibbon KA, Walker CJ, Willan AR. A program to enhance clinical use of MEDLINE. A randomized controlled trial. Online J Curr Clin Trials 1993; Doc No. 56.
21. Jaeschke R, Guyatt G, Sackett DL. Users' guides to the medical literature. III. How to use an article about a diagnostic test. A. Are the results of the study valid? Evidence-Based Medicine Working Group. J Am Med Assoc 1994;271:389–91.
22. Jaeschke R, Guyatt GH, Sackett DL. Users' guides to the medical literature. III. How to use an article about a diagnostic test. B. What are the results and will they help me in caring for my patients? The Evidence-Based Medicine Working Group. J Am Med Assoc 1994;271:703–7.
23. Hunt DL, Jaeschke R, McKibbon KA. Users' guides to the medical literature: XXI. Using electronic health information resources in evidence-based practice. Evidence-Based Medicine Working Group. J Am Med Assoc 2000;283:1875–9.
24. Cochrane Methods Group on Systematic Review of Screening and Diagnostic Tests: Recommended methods, updated 6 June 1996. http://www.cochrane. org/cochrane/sadtdoc1.htm
25. Wilczynski NL, McKibbon KA, Haynes RB. Enhancing retrieval of best evidence for health care from bibliographic databases: calibration of the hand search of the literature. Medinfo 2001;10(Pt 1):390–3.
26. McKibbon KA, Haynes RB, Dilks CJ, Ramsden MF, Ryan NC, Baker L, et al. How good are clinical MEDLINE searches? A comparative study of clinical end-user and librarian searches. Comput Biomed Res 1990;23:583–93.
27. Wilczynski NL, Walker CJ, McKibbon KA, Haynes RB. Preliminary assessment of the effect of more informative (structured) abstracts on citation retrieval from MEDLINE. Medinfo 1995;8 Pt 2:1457–61.
28. Wilczynski NL, Walker CJ, McKibbon KA, Haynes RB. Reasons for the loss of sensitivity and specificity of methodologic MeSH terms and text words in MEDLINE. Proc Annu Symp Comput Appl Med Care 1995:436–40.
29. Wilczynski NL, Walker CJ, McKibbon KA, Haynes RB. Quantitative comparison of pre-explosions and subheadings with methodologic search terms in MEDLINE. Proc Annu Symp Comput Appl Med Care 1994:905–9.
30. van der Weijden T, IJzermans CJ, Dinant GJ, van Duijn NP, de Vet R, Buntinx F. Identifying relevant diagnostic studies in MEDLINE. The diagnostic value of the erythrocyte sedimentation rate (ESR) and dipstick as an example. Fam Pract 1997;14:204–8.
31. Shojania K, Bero L. Taking advantage of the explosion of systematic reviews: an efficient MEDLINE search strategy. Eff Clin Pract 2001;4:157–62.

7

Analysis and Presentation of Data

James C. Boyd and Jonathan J. Deeks

Earlier chapters have considered principles of evidence-based medicine in relation to laboratory testing and how measures of outcome can be used to demonstrate the effectiveness of a diagnostic test. In this chapter, approaches to the analysis and presentation of data derived from studies on the diagnostic accuracy of tests are examined. Approaches are presented only for studies in which diagnostic testing results are binary (positive or negative). The reasons for heterogeneity of results between studies will be categorized, and statistical methods for combining results across studies are discussed.

The diagnosis of disease or the assessment of disease prognosis in medical practice often involves the performance of a diagnostic test. All diagnostic and prognostic testing is associated with some amount of uncertainty that can be subdivided into at least two components:

- imprecision of the diagnostic test itself
- inaccuracy in the interpretation of the diagnostic test

The ongoing evolution of new, more robust analytical methods and increased monitoring of quality control are reducing uncertainty related to the first cause. However, the reduction of uncertainty associated with the second cause can only occur with the development of more reliable and objective testing modalities and better methods for assessing the diagnostic value of these modalities. Careful studies are necessary to evaluate the clinical diagnostic utility of new potential biochemical markers accompanied by sound approaches for optimizing the information obtained from such studies. This chapter will focus on the statistical and data-handling approaches that may be employed in studies of diagnostic accuracy.

STUDIES OF DIAGNOSTIC ACCURACY

Depending upon what measurement scale is utilized for a given marker, potential biochemical markers may be classified as categorical or continuous-valued. Categorical markers are most frequently expressed in terms of two results (present or absent), although some categorical markers use an ordinal scale with three or more possible results (e.g., 1+, 2+, 3+, etc.). Continuous-valued markers can be converted to categorical tests using diagnostic thresholds. Any values equal to or above the diagnostic threshold are expressed as, for example, "positive," and values below the limit as "negative." Because there may be error in the determination of continuous-valued results, it is also common to define an "indeterminate zone" around the diagnostic threshold and to assign a third label of "indeterminate" to any result falling in that zone. In addition, as results that are more extreme in both directions are often more diagnostic, there are benefits of using multiple diagnostic thresholds to produce an ordinal categorization of study results.

Since frequent reference will be made to "diseased" versus "nondiseased" patient categories, or equivalently, to the "presence" or "absence" of disease, it is important to define these terms in the context of this chapter. Patients in the "diseased" category are those who have a specific target disorder whose diagnosis is directly related to application of a given diagnostic test. Patients in the "nondiseased" or the "absence of disease" category do not have the target disorder, but they may have other diseases with similar clinical presentations to the target disorder.

The goal of an evaluation study is to establish whether there is a relationship between the marker test result and some clinically defined endpoint (e.g., presence or absence of a disease, good or bad prognosis, suitable versus unsuitable for treatment). The strength of any relationship discovered must be evaluated to establish the utility of the marker in predicting disease or outcome in the individual patient. It will be assumed here that the clinical outcome category (disease versus nondisease, good versus bad prognosis, suitable versus unsuitable for treatment) can be accurately assessed by some independent criterion (a so-called reference standard or "gold standard").

The strength of any relationship discovered is used to characterize the utility of the marker in its specific application. Sackett et al. (1) reviewed potential applications of laboratory tests. Table 1 in Chapter 2 of this volume lists various applications for laboratory tests in decision making. Because tests are not always used for decision-making purposes alone (e.g., they may also be used in risk assessment, in epidemiologic studies, or for research), their evaluation must be tailored to their intended application. This chapter will not cover specialized test evaluation approaches for the latter cases, but it will consider the most common study designs and statistical approaches for test evaluation in the context of clinical decision making where there are two clear alternatives.

SUMMARY MEASURES OF DIAGNOSTIC ACCURACY

Several statistical indices have been defined to aid in the evaluation of qualitative binary tests or continuous-valued tests with defined diagnostic thresholds. Yerushalmy (2) introduced *sensitivity* and *specificity* as statistical indices of the accuracy of a diagnostic test. The sensitivity of a test is defined as its capability to make a correct (positive) diagnosis in patients who have the target disease, whereas the specificity of the test is defined as its capability to make a correct (negative) diagnosis in patients who do not have the target disease. Sensitivity and specificity are expressed either as percentages or proportions. These concepts are best appreciated by referring to a 2 × 2 table (Table 1). In this table, the column labels refer to the patients' true diagnosis and the row labels refer to the result of the test. The cells indicate whether the patients' diagnosis has been correctly or falsely predicted by the test. The sensitivity of the test is provided by the number of true positive results divided by the total number of cases with a confirmed presence of the disease, TP/(TP + FN). The specificity of the test is the number of true negative cases divided by the total number of cases with confirmed absence of the disease, TN/(TN + FP). The pattern of sensitivities and specificities observed when the performance of a test is evaluated at several diagnostic thresholds depict the *receiver operating characteristic (ROC)* curve (*see* accompanying box and Figure 1). For any of these measures to be useful, the underlying cases in the diseased and nondiseased populations must be carefully chosen to have an appropriately representative clinical spectrum (that is, representative of those patients in whom the test will be used in clinical practice including patients with other conditions within the differential diagnosis of the condition in question), with match-

Table 1
A 2 × 2 contingency table as used in studies of test diagnostic accuracy

	Disease present	Disease absent	Total
Test positive	TP	FP	TP + FP
Test negative	FN	TN	FN + TN
Total	TP + FN	FP + TN	TP + FP + FN + TN

TP, true positive; FP, false positive; FN, false negative; and TN, true negative.

Receiver Operating Characteristic (ROC) Curves

ROC curves are used to show the pattern of sensitivities and specificities observed when the performance of a diagnostic test is evaluated at several different diagnostic thresholds.

An ROC curve from a study of the detection of pulmonary embolism by D-dimer assay is shown in Figure 1. Patients with pulmonary embolism are likely to have increased concentrations of D-dimer due to the breakdown of fibrin in blood clots, whereas patients without pulmonary embolism are less likely to have increased concentrations of D-dimer. This pattern of results is seen in Figure 1, with the 500-μg/L threshold showing high sensitivity (0.97), but poor specificity (0.5) and the 1000-μg/L threshold showing lower sensitivity (0.85), but higher specificity (0.72).

The overall diagnostic performance of a test can be judged by measuring the area under the curve. Poor tests have ROC curves close to the diagonal (sensitivity = 1 – specificity). The ROC curve for excellent tests would rise steeply and pass close to the top left-hand corner, where both the sensitivity and specificity are 1. Summary ROC (SROC) curves are used in systematic reviews to display the results of a set of studies, the sensitivity and specificity from each study being plotted as a separate point in the ROC space.

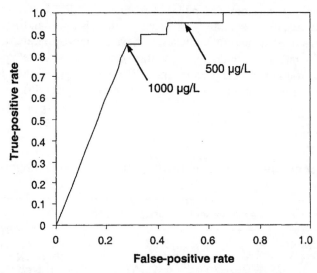

Figure 1 Receiver operating characteristic (ROC) curve of D-dimer for detecting pulmonary embolism in outpatients [adapted from (3)].

ing of age and sex composition and other clinical variables. Guidelines to ensure appropriate case selection will be covered later in this chapter.

The positive and negative *predictive values* (PV+ and PV−, respectively) for a diagnostic test are conditional probabilities first defined by Vecchio (4) and popularized in laboratory medicine by Galen and Gambino (5). PV+ expresses the probability that a patient has a target disease given that the test result is positive [TP/(TP + FP)] and PV− expresses the probability that a patient does not have the target disease given that the test result is negative [TN/(TN + FN)]. PV+ and PV− are known to depend upon the prevalence of disease in the patient population being examined. Although the sensitivity and specificity of a test may be high, the performance of the test as measured by the predictive value of a positive may be poor (low positive predictive value) when the disease prevalence is low in the population being tested. This dependence of predictive value on disease prevalence has made it difficult to transfer results from evaluation studies directly into clinical practice, as it is unlikely that the prevalence in clinical practice will match that observed in the study. This problem is particularly acute when patients with and without the target condition are sampled separately in the evaluation study.

The *likelihood ratio* of a test value (x) for analyte X is written L(X = x), or simply L(x), and is defined (6) as:

$$L(x) = \frac{\text{prob } (X = x | \text{Disease})}{\text{prob } (X = x | \text{No Disease})}$$

Likelihood ratios state how many times more likely particular test results are in patients with disease than in those without disease. For example, if the likelihood ratio is 10 for a positive test result, the probability of having a positive result in the diseased population is 10 times the probability in the nondiseased population. Likewise, if the likelihood ratio is 0.01 for a negative result, the probability of having a negative result in the diseased population is one-hundredth that of having a negative result in the nondiseased population. Thus, the farther a likelihood ratio deviates from a value of 1 (equal probabilities in the diseased and nondiseased populations), the more informative the test result corresponding to that likelihood ratio becomes. Negative likelihood ratios below 0.1 and positive likelihood ratios above 10 have been noted as providing convincing diagnostic evidence, whereas those below 0.2 or above 5 give strong diagnostic evidence (7). However, these guideline figures will not apply when pretest suspicions of disease are very high or very low. In these situations, more extreme negative or positive likelihood ratios will be needed, respectively, to rule-out or rule-in diagnoses.

Considering the special case of a binary test where x may take on only two values—plus or minus—then:

$$L(+) = \frac{\text{prob. positive result in patients with disease}}{\text{prob. positive result in patients without disease}} = \frac{\text{sensitivity}}{1 - \text{specificity}}$$

$$L(-) = \frac{\text{prob. negative result in patient with disease}}{\text{prob. negative result in patient without disease}} = \frac{1 - \text{sensitivity}}{\text{specificity}}$$

Unlike sensitivity and specificity, likelihood ratios can be used for tests that report more than two outcome categories. Each test result will have its own likelihood ratio. Likelihood ratios are therefore very useful for describing diagnostic accuracy for ordinal test scales and for continuous test results that have been categorized into more than two groups.

With use of the Bayes theorem, likelihood ratios can be directly applied to derive probabilistic statements regarding the likelihood of disease in an individual (6, 8). An example of this concept as applied to the D-dimer assay is shown in the accompanying box and Figure 2.

Due to the nonindependence of the test results, difficulties commonly

---

Likelihood Ratios

Likelihood ratios allow computation of posttest probabilities using Bayes theorem (6, 8) and the following formula:

Posttest odds = pretest odds × likelihood ratio

If the rate of pulmonary embolism in the outpatient population is correctly reflected by the 11 studies considered by Brown et al. (9) as being 28%, then the pretest odds are:

Pretest odds = prevalence/(1 − prevalence) = 0.28/0.72 = 0.39

Applying Bayes theorem to the pooled negative likelihood ratio:

Posttest odds = pretest odds × negative likelihood ratio
= 0.39 × 0.11 = 0.043

Converting posttest odds to posttest probability:

Posttest probability = posttest odds/(1 + posttest odds)
= 0.043/(1 + 0.043) = 0.041

Thus, only about 4% of patients with a D-dimer result less than 500 µg/L will have a diagnosis of pulmonary embolism. Calculations like this one are simplified by use of a Fagan pretest/posttest probability nomogram (Figure 2) (10).

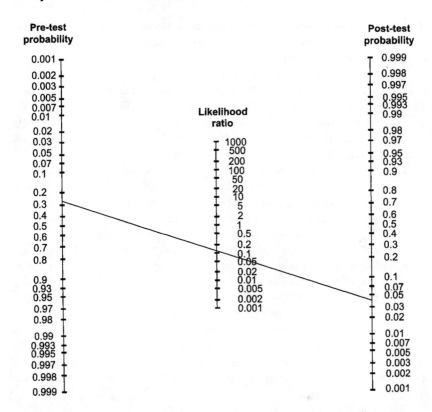

Figure 2 Pretest/posttest probability nomogram [after Fagan (10)]. To determine posttest probability, draw a line starting at the pretest probability value, continuing through the likelihood ratio for the diagnostic test. Extending the line until it intersects the right-hand-most axis will provide the posttest probability. A line has been drawn to depict the example described in the likelihood ratios box.

arise when trying to apply the Bayes theorem to update pretest probabilities using the results of several tests. Two approaches have been promoted to make allowance for the multivariate correlations between test results.

Spiegelhalter and Knill-Jones (11) described a two-stage method in which logistic regression is used to calculate shrinkage factors for individual test likelihood ratios, which account to some degree for the nonindependence of the diagnostic information contained in different tests. The approach only works for categorical test results.

Alternatively, Albert (6) described an approach by which the likelihood ratio for a combination of test results can be estimated using logistic regression. While the contributions of individual tests to the final likelihood ratios cannot be discerned, the approach allows overall likelihood ratios for all possible combinations of test results to be deduced. The Albert model also allows inclusion of continuous test results dependent on assumptions being made about linearity.

The derivation of both models uses the data from a diagnostic accuracy study. Using as a "training set" the test values from each person in a group of patients with and without the disease, logistic regression analysis can be applied to derive maximum likelihood estimates for the likelihood ratios. It is commonly recommended that the performance of models produced using these approaches is validated in new data sets.

The *diagnostic odds ratio (DOR)* expresses the odds of positive test results in patients with disease compared with the odds of positive test results in those without disease $[L(+)/L(-) = (TP \times TN)/(FP \times FN)]$. Unlike the other statistics presented so far (sensitivity, specificity, and likelihood ratios), the diagnostic odds ratio summarizes the accuracy of a test as a single value, which makes it well suited for use in meta-analysis. Where a given test has been assessed at different thresholds in multiple studies, it is possible that each of the studies will yield the same diagnostic odds ratio despite having different sensitivities and specificities. This will occur if the ROC plot is symmetrical, which will only occur if the variability of test results in patients with the target disease is the same as the variability in those without the target disease. Thus, a symmetrical ROC plot would argue strongly for the use of the DOR when combining the results from several studies in a systematic review. Unfortunately, in practice, ROC plots are not always found to be symmetrical.

META-ANALYSIS

Meta-analysis is undertaken to summarize the results of multiple studies addressing a single research issue. Meta-analysis is used as a method of data analysis during the performance of a systematic review, and is routinely used to evaluate the effects of therapies. It is particularly useful when:

- there are conflicting results among a set of studies, some of which have large sample sizes [e.g., the role of magnesium infusion in the treatment of myocardial infarction (12)], and
- there are inconsistently positive findings in a set of studies, none of which has large sample sizes [e.g., the role of adjuvant tamoxifen in early breast cancer first became apparent after a systematic review of all randomized trials of hormonal therapy or chemotherapy for resectable breast cancer as collated by the The Early Breast Cancer Trialists' Collaborative Group (13)].

In the first case, an analysis of a set of studies that investigates differences in research design may lead to explanations of the conflicting results.

In the second case, combining the results of several studies may give sufficient sample size and power to definitively answer the question at hand.

Similarly meta-analysis of studies of test accuracy involves the computation of a weighted average of individual study results, which can improve the precision of estimates of test accuracy and reveal between study differences that impact on test performance. As test accuracy is usually summarized by pairs of statistics rather than single statistics, and heterogeneity between study results is commonly encountered, statistical methods are more complicated than for meta-analysis of results of randomized controlled trials.

POOLING SUMMARY STATISTICS IN STUDIES OF DIAGNOSTIC ACCURACY

The first stage in any analysis should be to plot the individual study results. Two types of graphs can be used. Forest plots of test sensitivity and specificity display individual study results with associated confidence intervals (14). The consistency of each statistic can be gauged from the overlap of the individual confidence intervals. (Similar plots can be used to depict positive and negative likelihood ratios.) Plotting sensitivity against 1 − specificity (as for an ROC plot) will depict the heterogeneity by the scatter of points. From such a graph it is sometimes possible to discern whether there is a relationship between the heterogeneity in sensitivities and the heterogeneity in specificities.

There are two commonly encountered approaches to pooling results of diagnostic accuracy studies. The first analytical approach separately pools results of test sensitivities and then specificities, or positive likelihood ratios and then negative likelihood ratios. The attraction of this method is that it yields average values of these statistics, which are then usable in deciding clinical management dependent on test results. Methods for pooling these summaries and testing for heterogeneity are detailed in Deeks (15). If there is heterogeneity in the values that are being pooled, these summaries will be misleading and should not be used.

However, the graphical display in an ROC plot and tests for heterogeneity may identify that although points are scattered across the plot, there are particular summary statistics that are not affected by heterogeneity. For example, it is possible that while there is heterogeneity in sensitivities, specificities are reasonably constant, or negative likelihood ratios are constant whereas positive likelihood ratios vary. Thus, it may be possible in many circumstances to make useful conclusions about one dimension of test accuracy while noting that the alternate dimension is highly variable. Such partial information may be of clinical value in knowing that certain test results can be used to rule out or rule in the target diagnosis. But there will also be diagnostic tests in which all dimensions of test accuracy are highly variable, when no reasonable estimate of average sensitivity, specificity, and likelihood ratios can be produced.

The second analytical approach attempts to model and therefore explain the observed heterogeneity in test accuracy. One potential source of heterogeneity that needs to be considered is that introduced by explicit or implicit differences in the test threshold. Irwig et al. (16) have shown an example and referenced several studies where pooling the results of sensitivity and specificity across diagnostic studies can lead to problems when different studies use different test thresholds. If one study uses a test threshold that gives exquisite sensitivity, typically the test specificity in that study will be low. If, on the other hand, another study requires higher specificity, then the test sensitivity will be low. This tradeoff in sensitivity versus specificity needs to be taken explicitly into account in any statistical method for combining results. Otherwise, combining the results of two studies with two different extremes of test thresholds may lead to summary measures that indicate the test is of absolutely no value (16).

Several different approaches to fitting such summary ROC curves have been developed (17, 18). The simplest approach proposed by Moses et al. (17) is based on summarizing test accuracy in each study as a diagnostic odds ratio and on noting whether the diagnostic odds ratio is related to the proportion of patients in the study receiving positive test results (which changes as a consequence of changing threshold). Situations in which there is no relationship between the diagnostic odds ratio and threshold produce symmetric summary ROC curves, while situations where there is a relationship produce asymmetric curves.

The approach that Moses et al. (17) use involves first calculating the logits of the true positive (sensitivity) and false positive (1 − specificity) rates:

$$\text{logit(sensitivity)} = \log[\text{sensitivity}/(1 - \text{sensitivity})]$$

$$\text{logit}(1 - \text{specificity}) = \log[(1 - \text{specificity})/\text{specificity}]$$

and then computing the difference and the sum of these two components. The difference yields the log diagnostic odds ratio:

$$\begin{aligned} D &= \text{logit(sensitivity)} - \text{logit}(1 - \text{specificity}) \\ &= \log[\text{odds(sensitivity)}/\text{odds}(1 - \text{specificity})] \\ &= \log(\text{DOR}) \end{aligned}$$

while the sum is a transformation of the number of patients receiving positive results, which is dependent on test threshold:

$$\begin{aligned} S &= \text{logit(sensitivity)} + \text{logit}(1 - \text{specificity}) \\ S &= \text{logit(true positive rate)} + \text{logit(false positive rate)}. \end{aligned}$$

The relationship between diagnostic accuracy and threshold is then investigated by fitting a linear regression between D and S, which yields the equation of the fitted line:

$$D = \alpha + \beta S$$

where: α = intercept – the log DOR when S = 0

β = parameter describing how log DOR varies with threshold

The value of α gives the log diagnostic odds ratio at the point on the summary ROC curve where sensitivity is equal to specificity. In some texts, this point is referred to as Q* (17). Irwig et al. (16) discuss various unweighted and weighted approaches to fitting the regression line.

A test of the significance of the slope parameter β tests whether there is a relationship between threshold and diagnostic odds ratio. If it is nonsignificant, it is common to assume that the diagnostic odds ratio is constant across the studies and compute the average diagnostic odds ratio using standard meta-analytical techniques (8).

The summary ROC curve can be computed by transforming the linear relationship between D and S back to ROC space:

$$\text{sensitivity} = \left[1 = e^{-\alpha/(1-\beta)} \cdot \left(\frac{\text{specificity}}{1 - \text{specificity}} \right)^{(1+\beta)/(1-\beta)} \right]^{-1}$$

An example of the application of this approach is a study by Olatidoye et al. (19) who carried out a meta-analysis of studies of the diagnostic accuracy of troponin I and troponin T. Their study computed summary ROC's for the two markers and concluded that the two markers did not differ significantly in diagnostic accuracy. A drawback of the Moses approach to meta-analysis is that it is not possible to obtain point estimates of test sensitivity and specificity from the analysis, and therefore the usefulness of its clinical application is limited.

Extensions of the Moses approach allow differences in the diagnostic accuracy between tests to be examined by adding [0,1] indicator variables to the regression equation to indicate test type (20).

DEFICIENCIES IN STUDY DESIGN, ANALYSIS, AND REPORTING

Deficiencies in study design can affect the findings and conclusions of meta-analyses (20, 21). Reid et al. (22) found that only 18% of studies in the diagnostic testing literature published in five major journals over a 3-year-period observed more than five of seven methodological criteria. Lijmer et al. (23) found that studies with lower methodologic quality tended to overestimate the diagnostic performance of a test. To aid authors, reviewers and editors in the evaluation of future studies of diagnostic test accuracy, the STARD group has recently published guidelines for the publication of studies of test diagnostic accuracy (24, 25).

Lijmer et al. (20) pointed to several additional sources of variability and bias in clinical studies. Because disease status is seldom a true dichotomous classification, variation in the spectrum of disease from study to study can lead to varying estimates of sensitivity and specificity. Likewise, variations in the protocol for the reference test between studies can lead to additional heterogeneity. Where not all patients receive the reference standard, or where different reference standards are used for patients within the same study according to their experimental test results, study results may be affected by partial and differential verification bias. Lijmer et al. (20) suggest extensions to the model of Moses et al. (17) to evaluate the influence of methodological and/or clinical differences between studies.

In addition, when there are known or unknown subsets of data that have not been broken out in a meta-analysis, there is the possibility that the conclusions drawn using summary measures from the subsets may be different from those drawn from the overall dataset. For example, C-reactive protein concentrations are known to be increased in many individuals with an underlying autoimmune disease. Analysis of the value of C-reactive protein as a predictor of coronary artery disease in this patient subset will be vastly different from its diagnostic value determined in the population at large. In this case, breaking out the subgroup from the rest of the population helps to clarify the diagnostic value of the marker in each group. If individual data from studies are available, the meta-analysts may find that their analysis provides more accurate information regarding subgroups than analysis of aggregate measures from each study (26). For instance, different studies may define groups slightly differently, using different age thresholds to define "young" or "old" groups, or may not stratify their analysis by age at all. If the original individual patient data can be made available from each study, the meta-analyst can overcome this problem nicely. Otherwise, there is potential for biased and/or unusable data from studies reporting only summary measures. Increasingly, the original data from studies are becoming available. Some laboratory-based journals are beginning to encourage a similar practice in studies of diagnostic accuracy by offering to store datasets as supplementary files through their on-line journal web sites (27).

POTENTIAL SOURCES OF BIAS IN SYSTEMATIC REVIEWS OF TEST ACCURACY

Many factors can influence and/or bias the final results of a given study. Variation in these factors across studies of diagnostic test accuracy can lead to heterogeneity between studies. Since heterogeneous study results coming from noncomparable study designs can lead to erroneous conclusions, it is important to be aware of these factors and evaluate their degree of severity in a given study.

Egger and Smith (28) reviewed various factors that can lead to bias in meta-analysis of randomized controlled trials. These factors can be categorized as publication bias, language bias, indexing bias, and inclusion bias. These potential biases are likely to apply to studies of diagnostic accuracy, although at present there are no data on the extent of these effects.

Publication bias refers to the phenomenon that studies showing positive findings are more likely to be published than negative studies. Failure to find these unpublished studies can lead to overoptimistic estimates of treatment effect in drug studies, or of diagnostic value in test evaluation studies (28). Sutton et al. (29) estimated that approximately half of meta-analyses of randomized controlled trials may be affected by publication bias. Similar figures are not available in the diagnostic test evaluation literature. There is debate over the inclusion of findings from unpublished studies in meta-analyses (26). While their inclusion would substantially improve the accuracy of meta-analytic studies, many observers have been concerned that not all unpublished studies can be found by the meta-analyst, and that unpublished studies may not have been subjected to rigorous peer review. In addition, concerns have been expressed that interested parties (e.g., drug or diagnostic test manufacturers) might unduly influence which of the unpublished studies was included (e.g., those studies most favorable to their economic interests). Thus, it is currently recommended that the effects of unpublished studies be evaluated by performing separate meta-analysis, with and without the unpublished studies.

Language bias results from the fact that studies showing positive findings are more likely to be published in the leading journals that are usually published in English. They are also more likely to be cited and are more likely to be published repeatedly (28).

Indexing bias results from the effect that positive studies are more likely to be published in journals that are indexed (e.g., Medline) than negative studies.

Inclusion bias can result when the investigator performing the meta-analysis has knowledge of the results of a subset of potential studies to be included that may bias his or her selection of the inclusion criteria.

CASE STUDY: DETECTION OF PULMONARY EMBOLISM IN OUTPATIENTS USING THE D-DIMER ASSAY

Brown et al. (9) published a systematic review of 11 studies evaluating the diagnostic accuracy of the enzyme-linked immunosorbent assay D-dimer test in the diagnosis of pulmonary embolism in the adult emergency department population. All studies included in the review were prospective cohort designs and used the results of positive angiogram or autopsy results, high-probability V/Q scan, CT scan result positive for PE, or, positive lower extremity imaging study results as the reference standard for making a diagnosis of PE. Negative diagnosis was based upon a negative angiography result, normal or very low probability V/Q scan, or clinical followup documenting the absence of a thromboembolic event over a minimum of 3 months. All of the studies presented sensitivities and specificities of D-dimer for the diagnosis of pulmonary embolism. Several studies presented D-dimer results at multiple diagnostic thresholds. In such cases the authors used only the results obtained at a threshold of 500 µg/L (the most common diagnostic threshold). These 11 studies, selected from a total of 52 studies identified by a literature search, were the only ones that met prespecified inclusion criteria. All reviews and editorials were excluded. In addition, studies that did not consider outpatients separately from inpatients were excluded, as well as studies that did not meet the meta-analysis protocol definition of appropriate patient spectrum or reference standard. The case study presented here is based on reanalysis of the data from the 11 final selected studies in this review. Figure 3 shows the sensitivities and specificities for the 11 studies plotted as forest plots (14).

HETEROGENEITY IN STUDY RESULTS

The pattern of variability (heterogeneity) observed across studies plays a partial role in the choice of a meta-analytical method. Plotting the sensitivities and specificities from the studies as suggested by Moses et al. (17) allows graphical consideration of heterogeneity (Figure 3). Some variation of the results around a mean estimate can be expected by chance. However, other factors such as variation in study designs, heterogeneity of analytical methods used for diagnostic testing, and patient selection may increase the observed variability (30).

As already discussed, an important extra source of heterogeneity is variation introduced by changes in diagnostic threshold. Studies may use different thresholds to define positive and negative test results. Different investigators may deliberately have chosen to use different thresholds. For instance, to avoid large numbers of false-positive results when the prevalence of disease is very low in the population being studied, investigators may choose a more extreme threshold for the test. In addition, different thresholds may have been due to variation in test performance or test calibration from study to study.

If the heterogeneity between studies can be shown to be low, a single point on the ROC graph may be the best summary estimate of test perfor-

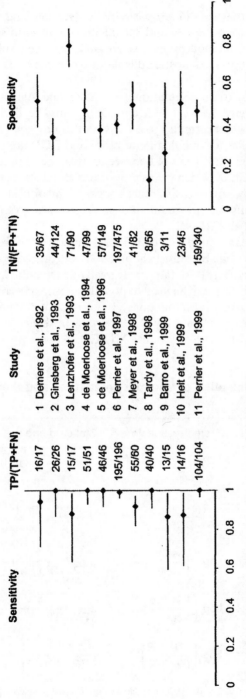

Figure 3 Forest plots of the sensitivities and specificities from 11 studies of D-dimer as reviewed by Brown et al. (9).

mance. Three approaches will be considered for summarizing the data. The first method pools sensitivities and specificities to develop summary estimates. The second method pools positive and negative likelihood ratios. The third method pools diagnostic odds ratios by the method of Moses et al. (17).

Preparatory to these calculations, estimates and standard errors for sensitivity, specificity, L(+), L(−), and DOR must be derived for each study. Table 2 provides formulas to assist with this process. Calculations to derive these statistics for the likelihood ratios and DOR are performed using log transformed data. Tests of homogeneity can be computed following the method of Cochran, which yields a chi-squared statistic computed as the weighted sum of the squared differences between the overall summary estimate and the results of individual studies. Details are given in Normand (31) and Deeks et al. (32).

The analyses can be undertaken in most standard software packages, as they use routinely available statistical functions. Software for meta-analysis of trials (33, 34) [such as RevMan, freely available from the Cochrane Collaboration website (35)] can be used to pool diagnostic odds ratios and likelihood ratios (using risk ratio functions), but not for meta-analysis of sensitivities, specificities and summary ROC curves. In this case study, results were pooled using the SAS procedure MIXED.

Table 2
Formulas for calculation of summary measures and their standard errors

Summary measure	From 2 × 2 table	Standard error
Sensitivity = sens	$\dfrac{TP}{TP+FN}$	$\sqrt{\dfrac{sens(1-sens)}{TP+FN}}$
Specificity = spec	$\dfrac{TN}{FP+TN}$	$\sqrt{\dfrac{spec(1-spec)}{FP+TN}}$
Log L(+)	$Log_e\left(\dfrac{sens}{1-spec}\right)$	$\sqrt{\dfrac{1}{TP}-\dfrac{1}{TP+FN}+\dfrac{1}{FP}-\dfrac{1}{FP+TN}}$
Log L(−)	$Log_e\left(\dfrac{1-sens}{spec}\right)$	$\sqrt{\dfrac{1}{FN}-\dfrac{1}{TP+FN}+\dfrac{1}{TN}-\dfrac{1}{FP+TN}}$
Log DOR	$Log_e\left(\dfrac{TN\times TP}{FP\times FN}\right)$	$\sqrt{\dfrac{1}{TP}+\dfrac{1}{FN}+\dfrac{1}{FP}+\dfrac{1}{TN}}$

Sens, sensitivity; spec, specificity; L(+), likelihood ratio of a positive; L(−), likelihood ratio of a negative; DOR, diagnostic odds ratio.

POOLING SENSITIVITIES AND SPECIFICITIES

The pooled estimate of mean specificity for D-dimer using a random effects model is 0.44 (95% confidence interval 0.35–0.54) and is depicted by the vertical line on the ROC plot in Figure 4A. The overall estimate of mean sensitivity is higher 0.96 (0.91–1.00). There is apparent heterogeneity in the study results depicted in Figure 4A. Although the study points lie reasonably close to the summary sensitivity (test of homogeneity, P = 0.149), the results for several studies lie some distance from the summary specificity (test of homogeneity P < 0.001).

Regardless of the sources of this heterogeneity, the overall high estimate and relative consistency of the mean sensitivity estimate for D-dimer suggest that a negative test result could be useful in ruling out pulmonary embolism. It is more difficult to draw any conclusions about test specificity. There is clearly a large range of specificities over the studies considered (0.14–0.79). The two lowest test specificities (0.14 and 0.27) occurred in studies with the oldest patients, but whether this is a real effect or simply coincidence is unclear.

POOLING LIKELIHOOD RATIOS

It is helpful to develop a graphical concept of likelihood ratios. The positive likelihood ratio is given by the slope of the straight line linking the bottom left-hand corner of the ROC plot to each study point. Similarly, the negative likelihood ratio is given by the slope of the straight line linking the top right-hand corner of the plot to each study point.

For the case study, the pooled estimate of the positive likelihood ratio was not particularly high, 1.74 (1.50–2.04), and the values varied significantly between the studies (test of homogeneity, P <0.001). In Figure 4B, it is clear that the slopes of the lines from the left-hand bottom corner to the study points vary considerably. Again it is debatable whether reporting the average value (the summary line for positive likelihood ratio) of such heterogeneous results is sensible, but it is unlikely that a positive test result could provide convincing evidence of the presence of pulmonary embolism as the positive likelihood ratios are all below 5 (data not shown).

Compared with the highly significant heterogeneity seen in positive likelihood ratios, the negative likelihood ratios displayed modest heterogeneity (test of homogeneity, P = 0.043), and provided more convincing evidence of the absence of pulmonary embolism, the pooled estimate being 0.11 (0.05–0.22). The slopes of the lines from the top right-hand corner of the ROC plot in Figure 4B to the study points are fairly similar and the summary line lies close to the results of most of the studies, suggesting that a measurement of D-dimer 500 µg/L or less can provide reasonably convincing evidence to rule out pulmonary embolus.

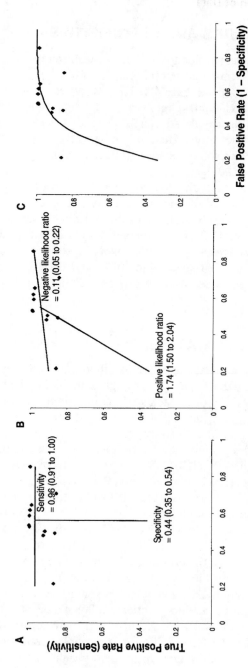

Figure 4 Plots of true-positive rates versus false-positive rates showing three approaches to meta-analysis of 11 studies of diagnostic accuracy of D-dimer testing for detection of pulmonary embolism. The 11 studies were those reviewed and described by Brown et al. (9). Results of the individual studies are plotted as diamonds. Fitted lines (A) show overall estimated sensitivity and specificity, (B) overall estimated positive and negative likelihood ratios, and (C) Moses-type summary ROC curve. Figures in parentheses are 95% confidence intervals for the summary estimates.

These results indicate that there is a high degree of heterogeneity in positive likelihood ratios, and less heterogeneity in negative likelihood ratios—similar to the findings observed by pooling sensitivities and specificities. However, pooled likelihood ratios have the advantage of being more easily interpreted and applied in clinical practice (*see* Likelihood Ratio box).

DIAGNOSTIC ODDS RATIOS AND SUMMARY ROC CURVES

In this case study, it is likely that some of the observed heterogeneity can be explained by a threshold effect, due to differences in thresholds or calibrations for the D-dimer assays from study to study. The estimate of the summary diagnostic odds ratio by a random effects model is 18.7 (8.7–40.2) and the nonsignificant test of homogeneity (P = 0.068) suggests that the points could have originated from the same symmetric ROC curve. With a symmetric ROC curve, each pair of sensitivity and specificity values is perfectly balanced by another pair in which the numerical values are identical, but reversed. If Table 2 in Deeks (9), for example, is consulted, a diagnostic odds ratio of 19 corresponds to a sensitivity of 0.5 and a specificity of 0.9, the reversed relationship, a sensitivity of 0.9 and a specificity of 0.5, and, by interpolation, a sensitivity of 0.81 and a specificity of 0.81.

However, if the summary ROC curve derived according to the approach of Moses et al. is plotted (Figure 4C), it is visibly nonsymmetric. The estimated values for the parameters α and β (95% confidence interval) were 1.6 (−0.2, 3.3) and 0.44 (0.003, 0.87), respectively. The slope, β, was found to be statistically significantly different from zero (P = 0.049) suggesting that log DOR has a relationship with test threshold for D-dimer. This relationship accounts for the nonsymmetric summary ROC curve and suggests that other factors beyond a threshold effect are influencing the diagnostic accuracy of D-dimer across these studies.

The odds ratio and the summary ROC curve do not allow derivation of a unique joint summary estimate of sensitivity and specificity: it is only possible to obtain a summary estimate of one value by specifying the value of the other. Due to this correspondence of the odds ratio to a list of linked sensitivities and specificities, the odds ratio does not allow the physician to calculate the probability of disease associated with a specific test outcome.

SUMMARY

Smith and Egger (26) have reviewed instances in which large randomized controlled trials reached similar conclusions to those published years earlier in systematic reviews of data. Smith and Egger conclude, however, based on numbers of literature citations, that clinicians appear to have relied on the results of the systematic reviews less frequently than they have the results of the randomized controlled trials. Data like these indicate that acceptance of meta-analysis by the medical community is still lagging. It may be that many practitioners view meta-analysis as a mysterious and complicated procedure. However, despite these complexities and the heterogeneity observed among studies, it is still possible to draw a simple and useful conclusion from the meta-analysis used for the example that D-dimer concentrations below 500 µg/L can be used effectively to rule out pulmonary embolism.

Although meta-analyses of studies of test diagnostic accuracy have potential to extract better conclusions by combining the information from several studies, each meta-analysis must be performed with appropriate data analytic methods and properly selected data sets. The commonly used data analytical approaches for studies of diagnostic accuracy were reviewed, and it was noted that the choice of pooling method critically depends on the nature and degree of heterogeneity found in the study results. While the summary ROC curve and diagnostic odds ratio methods appear to best deal with the existence of heterogeneity in study results, they do so at the cost of producing statistical summaries which are of little direct use in clinical practice.

It is also clear that for meta-analysis of studies of diagnostic accuracy to achieve acceptance, the quality of the underlying published data needs to be improved (22, 23). Many meta-analyses of diagnostic test accuracy have failed because there were insufficient published studies. Guidelines such as those developed by the STARD group (24, 25) should be helpful to authors designing and submitting studies for publication to ensure that these studies are reported in a nearly optimal fashion.

Laboratorians and those involved in the generation and clinical interpretation of diagnostic test data need to become more familiar with the principles of evidence-based medicine and meta-analysis. It has been the purpose of this chapter to explain the statistical data manipulations of meta-analysis clearly and make meta-analysis better understood and more easily accessible to the everyday practitioner. Equipped with such knowledge, the practitioner will better be able to interpret the results of meta-analytic studies and understand the strengths and limitations of such studies.

REFERENCES

1. Sackett DL, Haynes RB, Guyatt GH, Tugwell P. Clinical epidemiology; a basic science for clinical medicine, 2nd ed. Toronto: Little, Brown, 1991:1–441.
2. Yerushalmy J. Statistical problems in assessing methods of medical diagnosis, with special reference to X-ray techniques. Public Health Rep 1947;62:1432–49.
3. Schrecengost JE, LeGallo RD, Boyd JC, Moons KGM, Gonias SL, Bruns DE. Comparison of diagnostic accuracies in outpatients and hospitalized patients of

D-dimer testing for the evaluation of suspected pulmonary embolism. Clin Chem (in press).

4. Vecchio TJ. Predictive value of a single diagnostic test in unselected populations. N Engl J Med 1966;274:1171–3.

5. Galen RS, Gambino SR. Beyond normality: the predictive value and efficiency of medical diagnoses. New York, Wiley, 1975.

6. Albert A. On the use and computation of likelihood ratios in clinical chemistry. Clin Chem 1982;28:1113–9.

7. Jaeschke R, Guyatt GH, Sackett DL for the Evidence-Based Medicine Working Group. Users' guides to the medical literature. VI. How to use an article about a diagnostic test. B: What are the results and will they help me in caring for my patients? J Am Med Assoc 1994; 271:703–7.

8. Deeks JJ. Systematic reviews of evaluations of diagnostic and screening tests. Br Med J 2001;323:157–62.

9. Brown MD, Rowe BH, Reeves MJ, Bermingham JM, Goldhaber SZ. The accuracy of the enzyme-linked immunosorbent assay D-dimer test in the diagnosis of pulmonary embolism: a meta-analysis. Ann Emerg Med 2002;40:133–44.

10. Fagan TJ. Nomogram for Bayes theorem. N Engl J Med. 1975 Jul 31;293(5):257.

11. Spiegelhalter DJ, Knill-Jones RP. Statistical and knowledge-based approaches to clinical-decision support systems, with an application in gastroenterology. J R Stat Soc A 1984; 147: 35–77.

12. Seelig MS, Elin RJ. Is there a place for magnesium in the treatment of acute myocardial infarction? Am Heart J 1996;132:471–7.

13. Early Breast Cancer Trialists' Collaborative Group. Effects of adjuvant tamoxifen and of cytotoxic therapy on mortality in early breast cancer. An overview of 61 randomized trials among 28,896 women. N Engl J Med 1988; 319:1681–92.

14. Lewis S, Clarke M. Forest plots: trying to see the wood and the trees. Br Med J 2001;322:1479–80.

15. Deeks JJ. Systematic reviews of evaluations of diagnostic and screening tests. In: Egger M, Smith GD, Altman G, eds. Systematic reviews in health care: meta-analysis in context. 2nd ed. London: BMJ Books, 2001: 248–82.

16. Irwig L, Macaskill P, Glasziou P, Fahey M. Meta-analytic methods for diagnostic test accuracy. J Clin Epidemiol 1995;48:119–30.

17. Moses LE, Shapiro D, Littenberg B. Combining independent studies of a diagnostic test into a summary ROC curve: data-analytic approaches and some additional considerations. Statist Med 1993;12:1293–316.

18. Rutter CM, Gatsonis CA. A hierarchical regression approach to meta-analysis of diagnostic test accuracy evaluations. Statist Med 2001;20:2865–84.

19. Olatidoye AG, Wu AHB, Feng YJ, Waters D. Prognostic role of troponin T versus troponin I in unstable angina pectoris for cardiac events with meta-analysis comparing published studies. Am J Cardiol 1998; 81:1405–10.

20. Lijmer JG, Bossuyt PMM, Heisterkamp SH. Exploring sources of heterogeneity in systematic reviews of diagnostic tests. Statist Med 2002;21:1525–37.

21. Jüni P, Altman G, Egger M. Systematic reviews in health care. Assessing the quality of controlled clinical trials. Br Med J 2001;323:42–6.

22. Reid MC, Lachs MS, Feinstein AR. Use of methodological standards in diagnostic test research. Getting better but still not good. J Am Med Assoc 1995;274:645–51.

23. Lijmer JG, Mol BW, Heisterkamp S, Bosel GJ, Prins MH, van der Meulen JH, et al. Empirical evidence of design-related bias in studies of diagnostic tests. J Am Med Assoc 1999;282:1061–6.

24. Bossuyt PM, Reitsma JB, Bruns DE, Gatsonis CA, Glasziou PP, Irwig LM, et al. The STARD statement for reporting studies of diagnostic accuracy: explanation and elaboration. Clin Chem 2003;49(1):7–18.

25. Bossuyt PM, Reitsma JB, Bruns DE, Gatsonis CA, Glasziou, PP, Irwig LM, et al. Towards complete and accurate reporting of studies of diagnostic accuracy: the STARD initiative. Clin Chem 2003;49(1):1–6.

26. Smith GD, Egger M. Meta-analysis: unresolved issues and future developments. Br Med J 1998;316:221–5.

27. Clinical Chemistry, International Journal of Laboratory Medicine and Molecular Diagnostics. Information for Authors (Revised 01/24/2003). http://www.aacc.org/ccj/infoauth.pdf.

28. Egger M, Smith GD. Meta-analysis bias in location and selection of studies. Br Med J 1998;316:61–6.

29. Sutton AJ, Duval SJ, Tweedie RL, Abrams KR, Jones DR. Empirical assessment of effect of publication bias on meta-analyses. Br Med J 2000;320:1574–7.

30. Thompson SG. Why sources of heterogeneity in meta-analysis should be investigated. Br Med J 1994;309:1351–5.

31. Normand ST. Tutorial in Biostatistics. Meta-analysis: Formulating, evaluating, combining, and reporting. Statist Med 1999;18: 321–59.

32. Deeks JJ, Altman DG, Bradburn MJ Statistical methods for examining heterogeneity and combining results from several studies in meta-analysis. In: Egger M, Smith GD, Altman G, eds. Systematic reviews in health care: meta-analysis in context. 2nd ed. London: BMJ Books, 2001:285–312.

33. Egger M, Sterne JAC, Smith GD. Meta-analysis software. Br Med J 1998;316 electronic supplement available at: http://bmj.com/content/vol316/issue7126/fulltext/supplemental/221/index.shtml (accessed 3/28/03).

34. University of Leicester Department of Epidemiology and Public Health. Meta-analysis in practice—Information on available software. http://www.prw.le.ac.uk/epidemio/personal/ajs22/meta/ (accessed 3/28/03).

35. Review Manager (RevMan) [Computer program]. Version 4.1 for Windows. Oxford, England: The Cochrane Collaboration, 2000. Available at http://www.cochrane.org/cochrane/download.htm (accessed 3/28/03).

8

Systematic Reviews in Laboratory Medicine: Potentials, Principles, and Pitfalls

Andrea Rita Horvath, Daniel Pewsner, and Matthias Egger

Patients and society in general expect physicians to base their approach to a clinical problem on informed and rational diagnostic reasoning. This means that clinicians understand and readily apply the principles of diagnostic decision making, which includes estimating the pretest probability (prevalence) of the disease under consideration and applying appropriate information about the characteristics and discriminatory power of the diagnostic tests. Depending on the test characteristics a test result will modify the pretest probability to a larger or smaller degree to produce a posttest probability, which will then inform decisions on further testing, therapy, or both (1).

In laboratory medicine and elsewhere it has become simply impossible for the individual to read, critically evaluate, and synthesize the state of current knowledge, let alone keep updating this on a regular basis (2). Reviews have become essential tools for anybody who wants to keep up with the new evidence that is accumulating in his or her field of interest. Reviews are also required to identify areas where the available evidence is insufficient and further studies are required. However, since Mulrow (3) and Oxman and Guyatt (4) drew attention to the often poor quality of conventional, narrative reviews in the 1980s, it has become clear that conventional reviews can be an unreliable source of information. In response to this situation, there has been increasing focus on formal methods of systematically reviewing studies to produce explicitly formulated, reproducible, and up-to-date summaries of the effects of healthcare interventions (5–7). However, these efforts have so far been largely confined to the evaluation of efficacy and cost-effectiveness of therapeutic and preventive interventions. This is illustrated in Figure 1, which shows the yearly number of systematic reviews and

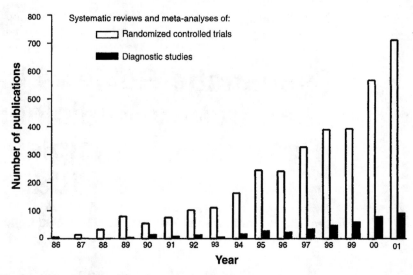

Figure 1 Number of publications concerning systematic reviews and meta-analysis 1986 to 2001 [Medline search using text word and medical subject (MESH) heading "meta-analysis" and text word "systematic review" combined with keywords denoting randomized controlled trials (open bars) and keywords denoting diagnostic test evaluation studies (solid bars).].

meta-analyses of randomized controlled trials and diagnostic test evaluation studies from 1986 to 2001.

If the ultimate purpose of laboratory medicine is improving clinical outcomes and prognosis, then the efficacy of diagnostic interventions and laboratory monitoring should ideally be assessed in randomized trials (8). Classic examples of assessing the clinical impact of a test (and therapeutic actions contingent on the test result) are randomized trials of screening. Unfortunately it is rarely feasible to assess the effect of diagnostic tests in randomized trials (a search in Medline combining publication type randomized controlled trial with the medical subject heading "laboratory techniques and procedures" returned just 28 citations in April 2003). In this chapter, systematic review and meta-analysis of test evaluation studies will be discussed; clearly, it is useful to systematically review and critically appraise the evidence that is available on the accuracy of tests for diseases or risk factors where effective interventions exist.

SYSTEMATIC REVIEW, OVERVIEW, OR META-ANALYSIS?

Several terms are used concurrently to describe the process of systematically reviewing and integrating research evidence, including "systematic review," "meta-analysis," "research synthesis," "overview," and "pooling." Chalmers and Altman (9) defined *systematic review* as a review that has been prepared using a systematic approach to minimizing biases and random errors which is documented in a materials and methods section. A systematic review may, or may not, include a meta-analysis; a statistical analysis of the results from independent studies, which generally aims to produce a single, overall estimate of a treatment's effect or a test's accuracy. The distinction between systematic review and meta-analysis is important because in principle it is always appropriate and desirable to systematically review a body of data, but it may sometimes be inappropriate or even misleading to statistically pool results from separate studies. Indeed, it is the impression of the authors that reviewers often find it hard to resist the temptation of combining studies when such meta-analysis is questionable or clearly inappropriate.

Traditional narrative reviews tend to be broader in range, often addressing the etiology, pathogenesis, diagnosis, clinical management, and the prognosis of a condition, whereas systematic reviews address a more narrow, specific question. Narrative reviews, editorials, and commentaries may express an opinion, speculate and hypothesize, and encourage new thinking and debate. Although narrative reviews tend to be subjective and are therefore more prone to bias and error than systematic reviews, they continue to have an important place in the medical literature (2, 10).

WHERE TO FIND SYSTEMATIC REVIEWS IN LABORATORY MEDICINE?

The number of systematic reviews of diagnostic studies has been slowly increasing in the last 10 years (Figure 1). One common source for finding high-quality systematic reviews is the Cochrane Library (http://www.up-date-software.com/cochrane/). However, only a few systematic reviews related to diagnostic procedures can be found in this database, as it mainly deals with therapeutic interventions. A recent issue (issue 4/2002) included 1519 reviews but only seven reviews of diagnostic procedures (0.5%), nine reviews of screening (0.6%), and 19 reviews of monitoring (1.3%). Several other databases have been established, such as the MEDION database, which contains more than 1000 references to reviews and methodological papers on diagnostic studies (available from berna.schouten@hag.unimaas.nl). The DARE database (http://agatha.york.ac.uk/darehp.htm), also published on the Cochrane Library, and the journals ACP Journal Club (http://hiru.mcmaster.ca/acpjc/default.htm) and Evidence-Based Medicine (http://www.bmjpg.com/template.cfm?name=specjou_be) include structured abstracts and commentaries of diagnostic reviews, which meet methodological standards. The database of the Committee on Evidence-Based

Laboratory Medicine of the International Federation of Clinical Chemistry and Laboratory Medicine consists of approximately 50 systematic reviews in clinical chemistry, some of which are critically appraised and followed by a brief summary (http://www.ckchl-mb.nl/ifcc). For a collection of evidence-based databases, the authors recommend using the database at the School for Health and Related Research (ScHARR) at University of Sheffield (http://www.sheffield.ac.uk/~scharr/ir/netting/).

STEPS IN CONDUCTING SYSTEMATIC REVIEWS

The following sections give an overview of the practical steps involved in systematic reviewing. These steps are summarized in Figure 2. This outline can only serve as an elementary introduction. Readers who want to perform systematic reviews should consult the other chapters in this book and other relevant resources (1, 5–7, 11). Although the focus is on clinical trials, the *Cochrane Reviewers' Handbook*, which can be downloaded free of charge from the internet, is also a useful source of guidance (12).

Developing a Protocol

Reviews should be viewed as observational studies of the evidence (13). The steps involved are similar to any other research undertaking: formulation of the question to be addressed, collection and analysis of the data, and interpretation of the results. Likewise, a detailed study protocol that clearly states the question to be addressed, the subgroups of interest, and the methods and criteria to be employed for identifying and selecting relevant studies and extracting and analyzing information should be written in advance. This is important to avoid bias being introduced by decisions that are influenced by the data. For example, studies that produced unexpected or undesired results may be excluded by post hoc changes to the inclusion criteria. Similarly, unplanned data-driven subgroup analyses are likely to produce spurious results. While every effort should be made to adhere to a predetermined protocol, it should be recognized that this is not always possible or appropriate. As a rule, changes in the protocol should be documented and reported. The protocols of Cochrane reviews are published in advance, which allows readers to assess to what extent the review process adhered to what was originally planned (14).

The review protocol ideally should be conceived by a group of reviewers with expertise both in the content area and the science of research synthesis. The composition of the review group depends on the question and the scope of the overview. In general, the panel of experts should represent the relevant professions that are involved in the problem area of the review. For example, if the review is about the use of urinary dipstick testing in primary care patients with symptoms of urinary tract infection, the review

---

1. Formulate review question (*see also* chapter 2)

■ Be as specific as possible

⇩

---

2. Define inclusion and exclusion criteria for studies

■ Clearly define experimental and reference test, disease or condition, patient characteristics and healthcare setting, outcome measures, and study designs

⇩

---

3. Locate candidate studies (*see also* chapter 6)

■ Develop search strategy in collaboration with librarian/information scientist
■ Consider checking of reference lists, the searching by hand of key journals, and communicating with experts

⇩

---

4. Select studies

■ Have eligibility criteria checked by two independent observers, resolve discrepancies by consensus
■ Keep log of excluded studies

⇩

---

5. Extract data and assess study quality (*see also* chapter 5)

■ Design and pilot data extraction form and quality checklist
■ Examine the presence of specific biases
■ Consider data extraction and quality assessment by two independent observers, resolve discrepancies by consensus

⇩

---

6. Analyze and present results (*see also* chapter 7)

■ Tabulate results from individual studies
■ Consider likelihood ratio plots (*see* Figure 3)
■ Examine between-study heterogeneity
■ Consider meta-analysis of all studies or subgroups of studies

⇩

---

7. Interpretation of data

■ Consider limitations
■ Consider strength of evidence
■ Consider economic implications
■ Consider implication for future research

Figure 2 Steps in the process of systematic reviewing [adapted from (13)].

group could consist of laboratory professionals, primary care physicians, urologists, and nurses. It is also helpful if an experienced librarian or information scientist and a biostatistician are part of the team. The protocol could be structured similar to Cochrane protocols:

• Cover sheet with information on the review group
• Background section

- Study question (*see also* chapter 2)
- Definition of experimental diagnostic test(s)
- Definition of condition(s), reference test(s), and patient population(s)
- Inclusion and exclusion criteria for studies (for example, reviewers may want to exclude diagnostic case-control studies—*see also* chapter 5)
- Search strategy (*see also* chapter 6)
- Assessment of study quality (*see also* chapter 5)
- Data extraction
- Statistical analysis and summary measures (*see also* chapter 7)

Formulating the Question

A clearly defined question is at the heart of any systematic review and is essential for guiding the review process, including strategies for locating and selecting studies, for critically appraising their relevance and validity, and for a priori defining analyses of between-study heterogeneity.

The question should clearly specify the type of laboratory test, the disease or condition, and the settings of care that are of interest. In addition, the types of studies that are relevant to answering the question should be specified.

What Type of Test?

The test whose performance is reviewed should be clinically relevant to current practice. It should be clearly defined, with detailed technical information if appropriate. The performance of new (and often expensive) tests may often be of particular interest. This test may be compared to other (older) tests in the same review. For example, Balk et al. (15) reviewed and compared the accuracy of biomarkers to diagnose acute cardiac ischemia in the emergency department, from creatine kinase to troponin I and T.

What Type of Reference Test?

Pragmatic considerations often limit the choice of an ideal "gold standard" which means that studies which may suffer from verification biases (*see* accompanying box for an overview of the biases that threaten studies of diagnostic accuracy) will have to be included in the review. For example, the "test of time" often plays an important role as a second reference standard. The reference tests should be clearly defined in the protocol. This inclusion will also facilitate the development of the appropriate search strategies for study retrieval.

What Type of Outcome Measure?

As already mentioned, evaluations should ideally employ the randomized controlled trial design, with "hard" clinical outcomes. This is, however,

> **Common Biases Threatening Diagnostic Test Evaluation Studies**
>
> **Spectrum bias:** Can be introduced when a test is evaluated in a study population, which is not representative for the settings where the test will be used. The classical example is the "diagnostic case-control study" when a group of patients with known disease is compared to individuals known to be free of the disease. In this situation, patients with unclear or borderline conditions and conditions mimicking the target disease are by definition excluded. This can lead to gross exaggeration of test accuracy (16).
>
> **Bias due to inappropriate reference test:** If the reference test used does not correspond to the best available test (gold standard), test accuracy will be underestimated. The degree of underestimation depends on the prevalence of the target condition (17).
>
> **Review bias:** Occurs when the reference test is interpreted with knowledge of the result of the experimental test, or vice versa. This often leads to overestimation of test accuracy, especially if interpretation of test results is to some extent subjective (16).
>
> **Partial verification bias:** Not all patients with negative results of the experimental test are subjected to the reference test. Some patients are either excluded or considered true negatives. This may lead to an overestimation of sensitivity and specificity or to an overestimation of sensitivity and underestimation of specificity (18).
>
> **Differential verification bias:** Not all patients with negative results of the experimental test are subjected to the (often invasive) gold standard test but undergo a different (less invasive) reference test. This may again lead to overestimation of test accuracy (16, 18).
>
> **Incorporation bias:** A type of verification bias where the experimental test result is combined with the result from the reference test and thus forms part of the gold standard. This will lead to an overestimation of test accuracy because experimental and reference test are not independent (19).

rarely feasible, and most diagnostic test evaluation studies therefore focus on a measure of diagnostic accuracy (*see also* chapter 4). Such measures of test performance can be classified according to whether they measure global, overall test performance in a single value or assess specific aspects of performance (e.g., sensitivity or specificity). Specific measures will be influenced by the choice of the threshold that separates test positives from test negatives whereas global measures should be independent of the calibration of the test. Another important issue is whether a measure is influenced by the prevalence of the disease in question (conditional measures) or not (unconditional measures) (20).

Reviewers are advised to focus on unconditional measures of diagnostic accuracy, such as sensitivity, specificity, or likelihood ratios (specific measures) or the diagnostic odds ratio (global measure) (20). *Likelihood ratios* indicate how many times more likely a test result is to be expected in an individual with the target condition than in a person without the condition (21). They have a number of advantages:

- Likelihood ratios give direct information about the power of a test to rule in a disease (likelihood ratio of a positive test or positive likelihood ratio) or to rule out a disease (likelihood ratio of a negative test or negative likelihood ratio). Positive test results with ratios greater than 10 and negative test results with ratios less than 0.1 are generally clinically useful (21).
- Likelihood ratios allow the use of the Bayes theorem to directly calculate posttest probabilities from pretest probabilities. A user-friendly nomogram (22) is available for this purpose.
- In the case of continuous measurements, likelihood ratios can be calculated easily for multiple thresholds.

For these reasons, the presentation of likelihood ratios in systematic reviews of laboratory tests is recommended.

What Type of Disease?

The choice of the test is closely linked to defining the disease or condition of interest. The same test may be used in the diagnosis of different conditions but perform differently in these situations. For example, the diagnostic power of the C-reactive protein is excellent for endocarditis but of limited use in appendicitis (23, 24). Importantly, reviewers should not only define the disease but also the stage or stages of the disease they are interested in.

What Type of Patients?

It is crucial to define the population and setting of interest. Important variables that more often than not will influence the performance of a diagnostic test include the age and sex distribution, the presence or absence of comorbidities, and whether people live in the community, in nursing homes, attend primary care centers, or are hospitalized in secondary or tertiary care centers. There are strong arguments for not restricting the review to specific population characteristics or settings; the degree of variation in test performance that is observed will often provide useful information. Furthermore, the broader the range of study populations and settings, the more readers will find information that is relevant to their circumstances.

What Types of Study Design?

State-of-the-art evaluations of diagnostic tests are based on prospectively enrolled individuals, apply the same reference test to all participants and evaluate results blindly (*see also* chapter 5). Diagnostic case-control studies, studies that use different or inappropriate references tests, and studies that are ill reported tend to overestimate test performance (16) and some reviewers may decide to exclude test evaluations that do not meet a basic set of quality criteria. If the reviewers are more restrictive in their inclusion criteria for studies, they will be less likely to identify studies that are relevant to the question. Although reviewing studies that are unlikely to provide reliable data is a frustrating exercise, it is important to demonstrate that the evidence that is available on a particular test is inadequate and that further studies of high quality are required. The inclusion of studies that differ in methodological quality may also allow the empirical demonstration of bias (16). The inclusion of all studies that meet very basic inclusion criteria, followed by analyses grouping studies by quality, may thus often be the best strategy.

Laboratory testing is about modifying the pretest probability to produce a posttest probability. Knowledge of the pretest probability or prevalence of the suspected disease in the population of interest is therefore essential to the interpretation of test results. Estimates of pretest probability will be available from test evaluation studies; however, it may be useful to perform additional literature searches and to present a more comprehensive review of prevalence estimates for a wider range of populations and clinical settings (25).

Locating and Selecting Studies

It is beyond the scope of this chapter to go into the technical details of literature searches in the field of laboratory medicine, and the reader is referred to chapter 6. The identification of diagnostic studies for systematic review generally involves both electronic and manual searches. Manual searches may include the hand searching of key journals and the reviewing of reference lists and bibliographies of previous reviews, textbooks, and other relevant articles (26). Manual searches are an important tool when locating diagnostic studies. The effort should be focused on the journals that are most likely to publish diagnostic test studies. These journals can be identified in Medline (Table 1). It should not be surprising that journals from laboratory medicine occupy the top ranks on this list.

Unfortunately there is no single search term denoting diagnostic studies in electronic databases. The overlap in the coverage of journals between the most widely used databases, Medline and EMBASE, is estimated to be around 35% (27). The overlap of a particular search executed in both databases will of course vary from search to search. Searches of other bibliographic databases should also be considered. The frequency with which the term "sensitivity and specificity" occurs in a database gives some indication which databases contain the largest number of diagnostic test evaluation studies (Table 2). Medline and EMBASE lead this list.

Assessment of Study Quality

The careful appraisal of the methodological quality and of other study characteristics is an important component of systematic reviews (*see also* chap-

Table 1
List of journals that publish many diagnostic evaluation studies[a]

Rank	Number of articles 1996–2000	Journal
1	994	J-CHROMATOGR-B-BIOMED-SCI-APPL
2	920	J-CLIN-MICROBIOL
3	718	RADIOLOGY
4	573	CLIN-CHEM
5	543	J-CHROMATOGR-A
6	471	AM-J-CARDIOL
7	430	AJR-AM-J-ROENTGENOL
8	361	ANAL-BIOCHEM
9	310	J-NUCL-MED
10	308	J-AM-COLL-CARDIOL
11	306	J-UROL
12	301	LANCET
13	294	CHEST
14	290	CANCER
15	280	GASTROINTEST-ENDOSC
16	271	J-VIROL-METHODS
17	254	J-MAGN-RESON-IMAGING
18	253	ULTRASOUND-OBSTET-GYNECOL
19	251	J-PHARM-BIOMED-ANAL
20	243	EUR-HEART-J
21	239	OBSTET-GYNECOL
22	230	MAGN-RESON-MED
23	229	BMJ
24	218	AM-J-GASTROENTEROL
25	213	CIRCULATION
26	212	EUR-RESPIR-J
27	207	ANTICANCER-RES
28	204	AJNR-AM-J-NEURORADIOL
29	198	CRIT-CARE-MED
30	195	AM-HEART-J

[a]Results from search with the terms "sensitivity and specificity" in Medline 1996–2000.

ter 5). Relevant factors that need to be assessed relate both to the internal validity (avoidance of bias) and external validity (generalizability) of studies. The validity of a diagnostic evaluation study should not be confounded with the test accuracy or the test retest reliability which describes the property of a given test to produce consistent results when applied to the same study population at different time points.

The optimal design of diagnostic test evaluations is based on a prospective blind comparison of the experimental test and the reference test (gold

Table 2
Ranking of literature databases according to the number of diagnostic test evaluation studies indexed[a]

Database	Number of articles
Medline (from 1966)	97,133
EMBASE (from 1974)	39,996
Science citation index (from 1980)	29,058
BIOSIS previews (from 1970)	21,611
CANCERLIT (from 1967)	20,787
Nursing and allied health (from 1982)	2880
PSYCINFO (from 1887)	1727
Alternative and complementary medicine from (1985)	115

[a]Search in July 2001 with the term "sensitivity and specificity" in the search system DataStar, which includes more than 300 bibliographic databases.

standard) in a consecutive series of patients from a relevant, well-defined clinical population (16, 28, 29). The patient population should cover the whole spectrum of disease and should be representative of the patients to whom the experimental test will be applied in the future. There are several biases that are known to threaten the validity of diagnostic test evaluations, including spectrum bias, bias due to an inappropriate reference test, review bias, verification bias and incorporation bias (*see* accompanying box).

How should study quality be assessed? There are essentially two approaches: quality scales that produce summary scores and checklists that assess the components of quality deemed to be important, without calculating a summary score (30, 31). Some of these instruments tend to confuse the quality of reporting with the quality of the design and conduct of a study by evaluating whether something was reported, rather than whether it was done properly. In the field of clinical trials, there is evidence that summary scores may be misleading, even if based on relevant aspects of methodological quality, because of inappropriate weighting of the different items (32).

Based on previous work (33, 34), the authors developed the included checklist (*see* Appendix) that covers the following items:

- the target condition and description of the evaluated test,
- the selection of study participants,
- the description of the study population,
- the reference test, and
- the statistical analysis and presentation of results.

The checklist concludes with an overall assessment of the study and the likely presence of different biases. Readers are encouraged to develop their own instrument, tailored to the needs and circumstances of their review.

It is good practice in systematic reviews to involve two independent reviewers in any assessment of information that involves subjective interpretation. This allows for analysis of interobserver agreement. This principle also applies to the assessment of study quality. In case of conflicting interpretation, disagreement can be resolved by consensus or by involving a third observer. It is advisable to use a pilot sample of articles to ensure that the reviewers apply the validity criteria consistently.

Summarizing and Presenting Results

Once studies have been selected, critically appraised, and data extracted, the characteristics and results of included studies should be presented in tabular form. This table will typically include likelihood ratios, sensitivities, and specificities along with relevant study characteristics, such as key aspects of methodological quality, and characteristics of the study populations and settings. Results from each trial are usefully graphically displayed together with their confidence intervals in a forest plot (*see also* chapter 7), a form of presentation originally developed for clinical trials (35).

Positive and negative likelihood ratios can be displayed on the same graph. An example, adapted from a meta-analysis of studies of troponin T in the diagnosis of acute myocardial infarction in emergency departments (15), is shown in Figure 3. Each study is represented by a point on the right and left side of the vertical line. The point on the left corresponds to the estimate of the negative likelihood ratio, with the horizontal line representing its 95% confidence interval. Similarly, the point and horizontal line on the right correspond to the point estimate and 95% confidence interval of the positive likelihood ratio. The solid vertical line corresponds to a likelihood ratio of 1, which represents a test result that has no effect on the pretest probability. Finally, the diamonds at the bottom of the graph represent the combined likelihood ratios with their 95% confidence interval from meta-analysis. A logarithmic scale was used, which has a number of advantages (36). Most importantly, the value and its reciprocal, for example, 0.5 and 2, which represent negative and positive likelihood ratios of the same magnitude, will be equidistant from 1.0. Furthermore, positive and negative likelihood ratios will take up equal space on the graph and confidence intervals will be symmetrical around the point estimate.

Such likelihood ratio plots thus allow a rapid assessment of the estimates from different studies of the power of a given test result to rule a diagnosis in or out. In this example, determination of troponin T is more useful for ruling in myocardial infarction than for ruling the condition out. Also, it is clear that there is some, but not extreme, heterogeneity between studies, which could be due to differences in the patient populations tested, the quality of studies (which was generally low), or differences in diagnostic thresholds (15).

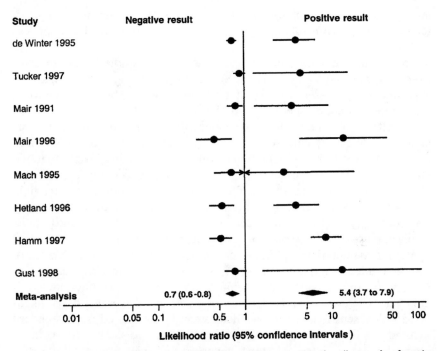

Figure 3 Likelihood ratio plot of eight studies of troponin T in the diagnosis of acute myocardial infarction. Key: The black points and horizontal line correspond to negative and positive likelihood ratios and 95% confidence intervals. The arrows indicate that confidence intervals extend beyond 1. The diamonds at the bottom of the graph represents the combined likelihood ratios from (random effects) meta-analysis. The results indicate that troponin T testing is more useful to rule the diagnosis in (combined likelihood ratio 5.4) than to rule it out (0.7). [Adapted from (15)].

Should Meta-Analysis Be Performed?

Systematic reviews of therapeutic and preventive interventions often use meta-analysis to statistically combine results from randomized controlled trials. This is appropriate for a set of trials of high methodological quality that examined the same intervention in comparable patient populations and clinical settings; each clinical trial will provide an unbiased estimate of the same underlying treatment effect (37). The variability that is observed between the trials can confidently be attributed to random variation and meta-analysis should therefore provide an equally unbiased estimate of the treatment effect, with an increase in the precision of this estimate. A fundamentally different situation arises in the case of observational studies, including test accuracy studies. Due to the effect of bias, threshold effects, and differences in the disease spectrum across study populations, studies may produce biased and heterogeneous estimates of test performance. Statistically combining a set of test evaluation studies may thus often provide estimates that are precise but biased and of uncertain applicability.

Meta-analysis should only be considered if the studies have recruited from clinically similar populations and clinical settings, used comparable experimental and reference tests, and are unlikely to be biased. Even when these criteria are met, there may still be such gross heterogeneity between the results of the studies that it is inappropriate to summarize the performance of a test in a single figure. In general, the thorough consideration of possible sources of heterogeneity may often provide more insight than the mechanistic calculation of an overall measure of test accuracy (38). The exploration of possible threshold effects is crucial in this context. Threshold effects are caused by different definitions of positivity in different studies. The possibility of a threshold effect must always be investigated, both statistically and graphically by plotting sensitivity against 1 – specificity (receiver operating characteristics plot, *see also* chapter 7) (38). In the absence of threshold effects (and other important sources of heterogeneity such as differences in study quality, patient characteristics, clinical settings, and variability in experimental and reference tests), weighted averages of the likelihood ratios, sensitivities, or specificities can be calculated using standard methods, as illustrated in Figure 3 (20). A detailed discussion of methodological issues in meta-analysis of diagnostic test evaluation studies is provided elsewhere (20, 38–40).

Interpreting and Discussing Results

The discussion section should be clearly structured, with a statement summarizing the principle findings at the beginning, and generally address the following points (41, 42):

- The strengths and weaknesses of the review, including an assessment of the probability of bias
- The strengths and weaknesses in relation to other reviews, if applicable
- The degree of between-study heterogeneity, and possible explanations for heterogeneity
- The applicability of the results to different populations and settings, taking into account current diagnostic strategies
- The implications for clinicians and policymakers, including considerations of trade-offs between the expected benefits, harms, and costs of using the test in question
- Unanswered questions and future research

A brief assessment of the methodological quality of component studies, with particular emphasis on the typical biases that affect diagnostic studies, and of publication bias and other reporting biases is an important part of the discussion section. If there is clear evidence of bias, and if sensitivity analyses show that this could seriously affect conclusions, then reviewers should not shrink from recommending that the evidence to date be disregarded (43).

In addition to identifying limitations of their review, reviewers should discuss potential sources of heterogeneity in results. Such heterogeneity should not only be seen as a problem in a review but also as an opportunity that may lead to additional insight. Are there identifiable factors that may cause the test performances to vary? As mentioned, these factors could include differences in test application and interpretation and other reasons for threshold effects and differences in the disease spectrum.

The discussion about applicability of results in different population settings will depend on knowledge of the particular circumstances. In addressing the applicability of the results of a review, reviewers should be cautious not to assume that their own circumstances, or the circumstances reflected in the included studies are necessarily the same as those of others (42).

Other types of evidence that may be important in interpreting the results of test evaluation studies include prevalence studies (these may be formally included in the review), but also studies on the performance of the same test in other diseases, or the performance of other tests in the same condition, as well as studies of physiological or biochemical processes (including animal studies) that are relevant in this context.

LIMITATIONS AND UNRESOLVED ISSUES

Despite the crucial importance of an appropriate use of diagnostic and screening tests in clinical decision making, the process of building a systematically assembled and critically appraised evidence base for the evaluation of diagnostic and screening interventions has only just started. Systematic reviews are always useful for summarizing the available evidence, evaluating the quality of published studies, and accounting for variation in findings between studies. However, both the potentials and limitations of systematic reviews in the assessment of diagnostic technologies in laboratory medicine are far less well defined than in the evaluation of efficacy and cost-effectiveness of therapeutic and preventive interventions.

Take, for example, publication bias and related biases in the dissemination of research findings. In the randomized controlled trials literature, the existence of these biases is well documented; publication bias can distort findings because trials with statistically significant results are more likely to get published, and more likely to be published without delay, than trials without significant results (44). Among published trials, those with significant results are more likely to get cited, and more likely to be published more than once which means that they will also be more likely to be identified and included in reviews. Are these biases important in laboratory medicine? Probably yes, but the evidence base is thin at present. A recent study demonstrated that smaller studies tend to report better test accuracy, which may be due to publication bias, but the authors concluded that more research is needed to clarify the mechanisms underlying this finding (45).

The decision to test and the interpretation of test results are usually judged in the context of other information. The evaluation of the performance of a diagnostic test should therefore ideally integrate data on disease prevalence, test characteristics, utilization, and the interdependence of several tests. The impact on decisions regarding further testing and therapy and effects on patient outcomes, taking into account costs and values, should also be considered. Faced with this Herculean task, reviewers appear to have settled for what is feasible; published systematic reviews and meta-analyses tend to be based on studies of a single test that was evaluated in isolation, which limits their usefulness and applicability. Furthermore, the rapid pace of innovations in diagnostic technology means that evaluation studies may be out of date when they are completed.

What evidence do clinicians need to practice evidence-based laboratory medicine and, in general, to improve diagnostic cost-effectiveness? The barriers to the optimal use and appropriate interpretation of test evaluation data in clinical practice are ill understood at present. Likelihood ratios and prediction rules are advocated to convert pretest probabilities of disease into posttest probabilities, which should overcome many of the cognitive biases that are known to affect diagnostic problem solving (46). Informal methods of opinion revision, however, continue to dominate in practice. More research is needed to examine the barriers to the optimal use and appropriate interpretation of test evaluation data in clinical practice.

The evidence base on diagnostic tests and pretest probabilities today is reminiscent of the situation that existed for efficacy and effectiveness of treatments in the 1980s. The authors have suggested that an international collaboration should be established and a Bayes Library of Diagnostic Studies and Reviews, which would mirror the Cochrane Library, be created in order to remedy this situation (22, 44). In light of the described difficulties, international debate is needed to define the best way forward, but surely the time is ripe for a systematically assembled evidence base to support laboratory medicine.

ACKNOWLEDGEMENTS

We are grateful to many colleagues and friends who have commented on previous drafts, shared material, and offered encouragement, including Markus Battaglia, Heiner Bucher, Fritz Grossenbacher, Christoph Minder, Doug Altman, Jürg Bleuer, Patrick Bossuyt, Iain Chalmers, Jon Deeks, Paul Dieppe, Paul Glasziou, Les Irwig, Peter Jüni, Jeroen Lijmer, Gerben ter Riet, and David Simel.

APPENDIX

Checklist for Critically Assessing Diagnostic Studies

1. Bibliographic reference of study	
Reference Manager Nr.	
1.1 Authors	
1.2 Title	
1.3 Journal, year	

2. Target condition and description of experimental test(s)	
2.1 What target condition was evaluated?	_____
2.2 What experimental test(s) was (were) evaluated?	_____
2.3 Have multiple cut-offs for the test been defined?	O yes O no
2.4 What were the cut-off values?	_____
2.5 Was information provided on intra- or interobserver variability?	O yes O no
2.6 Were technical performance characteristics of experimental test given?	O yes O no test method: analytical sensitivity: specificity: trueness: precision: other:
2.7 Did the interpretation of the test rely on subjective interpretation?	O yes O no
2.8 Give number of observers involved (give kappa statistics)	_____kappa_____ O not given
2.9 How was disagreement resolved?	_____

3. Recruitment of participants into the study	
3.1 How were participants selected for the study?	O consecutively O random sample O other, specify: _____
3.2 Was this a diagnostic case-control study?	O yes O no comment:
3.3 Were patients with unknown diagnosis prospectively recruited into the study or was the study retrospective?	O prospective O retrospective
3.4 Was the selection of patients influenced by the presence of risk factors, symptoms, or results of previous tests? Please specify more	O risk factors O symptoms O previous results comment:

Checklist for Critically Assessing Diagnostic Studies *(continued)*

4. Description of study population	
4.1 What was the age, sex, ethnic, and sociodemographic distribution of the study population?	Age: O mean ___ O range___O other, specify: _____ male – female: number: .._/._. or %:__/__.. ethnic:_____ Other (sociodemogr.):_____.
4.2 Were symptoms of the target condition described? 4.3 What symptoms were present? 4.4 How severe were these symptoms? Give scores or grading where appropriate.	O yes O no _____ _____ _____
4.5 What was the prevalence of comorbid conditions?	Condition:_____ prev:.___% Condition:_____ prev:___%
4.6 What setting is the study population most likely to represent:	O the general population (health survey, screening)? O primary care population? O referred population from well-defined catchment area? O ill-defined referred population?

5. Application of the reference test(s)	
5.1 What reference test(s) was (were) used?	_____
5.2 Was the reference standard applied to all or only a fraction of study participants?	O all individuals O fraction
5.3 Were other reference tests applied? Please specify.	O yes O no
5.4 If clinical evolution without therapy was one of the reference tests, how long were patients followed up?	time_____ O not mentioned
5.5. Has any treatment occurred between the time of application of the test and the reference test?	O yes O no
5.6 Was information provided on intra- or interobserver variability?	O yes O no
5.7 Were technical performance characteristics of reference test given?	O yes O no test method: analytical sensitivity: specificitity: trueness: precision: other:
5.8 Did the interpretation of the reference test rely on subjective interpretation?	O yes O no
5.9 Give number of observers involved? (give kappa statistics) 5.10 How was disagreement resolved?	_____kappa_____ O not given _____
5.11 Did the result of the experimental test influence the application of the reference test?	O yes O no O not mentioned
5.12 Did the presence or absence of signs or symptoms of the target disease influence the application of the reference test?	O yes O no O not mentioned

Checklist for Critically Assessing Diagnostic Studies *(continued)*

5.13 Were the results of the experimental test interpreted without knowledge of the reference test?	O yes O no O not mentioned
5.14 Were the results of the reference test interpreted without knowledge of the experimental test?	O yes O no O not mentioned
5.15 Was relevant clinical information available to assessor when evaluating experimental or reference tests?	O yes O no O not mentioned

6. Presentation of results and statistical analysis	
6.1 Number of patients eligible enrolled tested with experimental test tested with reference test analyzed excluded from analysis?	____ ____ ____ ____ ____ ____
6.2 What were the reasons for excluding patients from the analysis?	—————————— —
6.3 How many test results were determinate? 6.4 How many test results were indeterminate? 6.5 How were the latter dealt with in statistical analysis?	____ ____ _____
6.6 How were the results of test accuracy reported? Sensitivity? Confidence Interval (CI) Specificity? CI? Positive Likelihood Ratio? CI? Negative Likelihood Ratio? CI? Area under the ROC? CI? Diagnostic Odds Ratios (DORs)? CI? Other measures (PPV, NPV, accuracy, etc.)?	 sens: ___ % CI: _____ spec: ___ % CI: _____ LR+ve: ___ CI: _____ LR-ve: ___ CI: _____ area: ___ CI: _____ DOR: ___ CI: _____ _____
6.7 What were the results? Please complete 2x2 table(s) for all patients and relevant subgroups, give ROC-Graphs or other statistics with 95% Confidence Intervals	
6.8 What was the prevalence of the target disease overall and in clinically relevant subgroups?	Overall: ___ % Subgroups:_____

7. Overall assessment of study characteristics	
7.1 Compared to a similar setting of other studies, what is the prevalence of the target condition in this study?	O high O medium O low
7.2 What is the probability of <u>spectrum bias</u> in this study?	O high O medium O low O very low
7.3 What is the probability of <u>differential verification bias</u> in this study?	O high O medium O low O very low
7.4 What is the probability of <u>partial verification bias</u> in this study?	O high O medium O low O very low
7.5 What is the probability of <u>review bias</u> in this study?	O very high O high O medium O low

Checklist for Critically Assessing Diagnostic Studies *(continued)*

7.6. What is the probability of <u>incorporation bias</u> in this study?	O high O medium O low
7.7 Is the <u>choice of the reference test(s)</u> appropriate?	O yes O no other: _____
7.8. How likely do the descriptions of tests and populations allow reproducing the <u>study results</u>?	O high O medium O low

8. Decision	
Does this study meet basic quality criteria allowing for inclusion? *If no, specify why:*	

REFERENCES

1. Black EA, Bordley DR, Tape TG, Panzer RJ. Diagnostic strategies for common medical problems. Philadelphia: American College of Physicians, 1999.
2. Horton R. The information wars. Lancet 1999;353:164–5.
3. Mulrow CD. The medical review article: state of the science. Ann Intern Med 1987;106:485–8.
4. Oxman AD, Guyatt GH. Guidelines for reading literature reviews. Can Med Assoc J 1988;138:697–703.
5. Egger M, Smith GD, Altman DG. Systematic reviews in health care: Meta-analysis in context. London: BMJ Books, 2001.
6. Mulrow CD, Cook D. Systematic reviews: synthesis of best evidence for health care decisions. Philadelphia: American College of Physicians, 1998.
7. Glasziou P, Irwig L, Bain C, Colditz G. Systematic reviews in health care: a practical guide. Cambridge, UK: Cambridge University Press, 2001.
8. Bossuyt PM, Lijmer JG, Mol BW. Randomised comparisons of medical tests: sometimes invalid, not always efficient. Lancet 2000;356:1844–7.
9. Chalmers I, Altman D. Systematic reviews. London: BMJ Publishing Group, 1995.
10. Egger M, Ebrahim S, Smith GD. Where now for meta-analysis? Int J Epidemiol. 2002;31:1–5.
11. Knottnerus JA. The evidence base of clinical diagnosis. London: BMJ Publishing Group, 2002.
12. Clarke M, Oxman AD, eds. Cochrane reviewers' handbook 4.1.6 [updated January 2003]. http://www.cochrane.dk/cochrane/handbook/handbook.htm (accessed April 2003).
13. Egger M, Davey Smith G. Principles and procedures. In: Egger M, Smith GD, Altman DG, eds. Systematic reviews in health care: meta-analysis in context, London: BMJ Books, 2001.
14. Antes G, Oxman AD. The Cochrane collaboration. In: Egger M, Smith GD, Altman DG, eds. Systematic reviews in health care: meta-analysis in context,. London: BMJ Books, 2001:447–58.

15. Balk EM, Ioannidis JP, Salem D, Chew PW, Lau J. Accuracy of biomarkers to diagnose acute cardiac ischemia in the emergency department: a meta-analysis. Ann Emerg Med 2001;37:478–94.

16. Lijmer JG, Mol BW, Heisterkamp S, Bonsel GJ, Prins MH, van der Meulen JH, et al. Empirical evidence of design-related bias in studies of diagnostic tests. J Am Med Assoc 1999;282:1061–6.

17. Irwig L, Bossuyt P, Glasziou P, Gatsonis C, Lijmer J. Designing studies to ensure that estimates of test accuracy are transferable. Br Med J 2002;324:669–71.

18. Panzer RJ, Suchman AL, Griner PF. Workup bias in prediction research. Med Decis Making 1987;7:115–9.

19. Ransohoff DF, Feinstein AR. Problems of spectrum and bias in evaluating the efficacy of diagnostic tests. N Engl J Med 1978;299:926–30.

20. Deeks JJ. Systematic reviews of evaluations of diagnostic and screening tests. In: Egger M, Smith GD, Altman DG, eds. Systematic reviews in health care: metaanalysis in context,. London: BMJ Books, 2001:248–82.

21. Jaeschke R, Guyatt GH, Sackett DL. Users' guides to the medical literature. III. How to use an article about a diagnostic test. B. What are the results and will they help me in caring for my patients? J Am Med Assoc 1994;271:703–7.

22. Fagan TJ. Nomogram for Bayes theorem. N Engl J Med 1975;293:257.

23. Hogevik H, Olaison L, Andersson R, Alestig K. C-reactive protein is more sensitive than erythrocyte sedimentation rate for diagnosis of infective endocarditis. Infection 1997;25:82–5.

24. Andersson RE, Hugander AP, Ghazi SH, Ravn H, Offenbartl SK, Nystrom PO, et al. Diagnostic value of disease history, clinical presentation, and inflammatory parameters of appendicitis. World J Surg 1999;23:133–40.

25. Pewsner D, Bleuer JP, Jüni P, et al. Do we need a Bayes Collaboration? Proposal for a diagnostic database. 13th Cochrane Colloquium, Cape Town, South Africa, October 2000.

26. van der Weijden T, IJzermans CJ, Dinant GJ, van Duijn NP, de Vet R, Buntinx F. Identifying relevant diagnostic studies in MEDLINE. The diagnostic value of the erythrocyte sedimentation rate (ESR) and dipstick as an example. Fam Pract 1997;14:204–8.

27. Smith BJ, Darzins PJ, Quinn M, Heller RF. Modern methods of searching the medical literature. Med J Aust 1992;157:603–11.

28. Reid MC, Lachs MS, Feinstein AR. Use of methodological standards in diagnostic test research. Getting better but still not good. J Am Med Assoc 1995;274:645–51.

29. Jaeschke R, Guyatt GH, Sackett DL. Users' guides to the medical literature. III. How to use an article about a diagnostic test. A. Are the results of the study valid? J Am Med Assoc 1994;271:389–91.

30. Moher D, Jadad AR, Nichol G, Penman M, Tugwell P, Walsh S, et al. Assessing the quality of randomized controlled trials: an annotated bibliography of scales and checklists. Control Clin Trials 1995;16:62–73.

31. Moher D, Jadad AR, Tugwell P. Assessing the quality of randomized controlled trials. Current issues and future directions. Int J Technol Assess Hlth Care 1996;12:195–208.

32. Jüni P, Witschi A, Bloch R, Egger M. The hazards of scoring the quality of clinical trial for meta-analysis. J Am Med Assoc 1999;282:1054–60.

33. Arrivé L, Renard R, Carrat F, Belkacem A, Dahan H, Le Hir P, et al. A scale of methodological quality for clinical studies of radiologic examinations. Radiology 2000;217:69–74.
34. Bruns DE, Huth EJ, Magid E, Young DS. Toward a checklist for reporting of studies of diagnostic accuracy of medical tests. Clin Chem 2000;46:893–5.
35. Egger M, Smith GD, O'Rourke K. Rationale, potentials and promise of systematic reviews . In Egger M, Smith GD, Altman DG, eds. Systematic reviews in health care: meta-analysis in context. London: BMJ Books, 2001:23–42.
36. Galbraith R. A note on graphical presentation of estimated odds ratios from several clinical trials. Stat Med 1988;7:889–94.
37. Egger M, Schneider M, Davey Smith G. Spurious precision? Meta-analysis of observational studies. Br Med J 1998;316:140–5.
38. Lijmer JG, Bossuyt PM, Heisterkamp SH. Exploring sources of heterogeneity in systematic reviews of diagnostic tests. Stat Med 2002;21:1525–37.
39. Oosterhuis WP, Niessen RW, Bossuyt PM. The science of systematic reviewing studies of diagnostic tests. Clin Chem Lab Med 2000;38:577–88.
40. Irwig L, Tosteson AN, Gatsonis C, Leu J, Colditz G, Chalmers TC, et al. Guidelines for meta-analyses evaluating diagnostic tests. Ann Intern Med 1994;120:667–76.
41. Docherty M, Smith R. The case for structuring the discussion of scientific papers. Br Med J 1999;318:1224–5.
42. Clarke M, Oxman AD, eds. Interpreting results. Cochrane reviewers' handbook 4.1.6 [updated January 2003]; Section 4. http://www.cochrane.dk/cochrane/handbook/handbook.htm (accessed April 2003).
43. Sterne JA, Egger M, Smith GD. Systematic reviews in health care: Investigating and dealing with publication and other biases in meta-analysis. Br Med J 2001;323:101–5.
44. Egger M, Dickersin K, Davey Smith G. Problems and limitations in conducting systematic reviews. In: Egger M, Smith GD, Altman DG, eds. Systematic reviews in health care: meta-analysis in context. London: BMJ Books, 2001:43–68.
45. Song F, Khan KS, Dinnes J, Sutton AJ. Asymmetric funnel plots and publication bias in meta-analyses of diagnostic accuracy. Int J Epidemiol 2002;31:88–95.
46. Elstein AS, Schwartz A. Clinical problem solving and diagnostic decision making: a selective review of the cognitive research literature. In: Knottnerus JA, ed. The evidence base of clinical diagnosis. London: BMJ Publishing Group, 2002:179–95.
47. Straus SE. Reporting diagnostic tests. Br Med J 2003;326:3–4.

9

Economic Evaluation of Diagnostic Tests

Deborah A. Marshall and Bernie J. O'Brien

Diagnostic tests are an important tool of modern medicine, offering a means of improving population health by early identification of disease and targeted deployment of effective medicines and surgery. But, diagnostic tests also use healthcare resources, and cost considerations now form part of the evaluative hurdle for new diagnostic and therapeutic tools in many parts of the world (1–5). This chapter explores what evidence is needed to establish whether a diagnostic test is "cost effective" such that it can be said to offer good value for money. Extending beyond the operating characteristics and clinical utility of a test, this chapter examines how the costs and health consequences of a test should be measured to permit comparison with other programs that are competing for resources in a healthcare system. After introducing a general framework for the hierarchy of evidence related to diagnostic testing, the approaches to economic evaluation are reviewed with examples from the published literature. The framework of the chapter is a well-known 10-point checklist for critical appraisal of economic studies (6) to structure and illustrate the methods of evaluation with examples from the published literature. The chapter concludes by discussing some specific challenges that arise in the economic evaluation of diagnostic tests.

THE HIERARCHY OF EVIDENCE FOR DIAGNOSTIC TESTS

Fryback and Thornbury (7) presented a hierarchical framework for evaluative evidence in relation to diagnostic imaging. The framework is shown as an evidence pyramid in Figure 1. Movement up the pyramid represents progression from *efficacy* (probability that the test works under ideal conditions of use) at the lower levels, to *effectiveness* (probability that the test works under ordinary conditions of use) in the middle, to *efficiency*

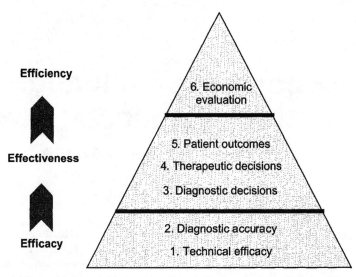

Figure 1 Hierarchial model for evaluation of diagnostic tests [adapted from (7)].

(the optimal use of limited healthcare resources) at the top levels. This conceptual framework applies equally well to both diagnostic imaging technologies and diagnostic laboratory tests. Guyatt et al. (8) applied a similar framework to computed tomography (CT) and magnetic resonance (MR) scanning, and Silverstein and Boland (9) applied it to case finding in ambulatory patient testing.

Diagnostic tests are most frequently evaluated at the lower levels (levels 1 and 2) of the pyramid which are concerned with the technical performance and diagnostic accuracy (sensitivity and specificity) of the diagnostic test. In the middle of the pyramid, levels 3, 4, and 5 concentrate on the impact of diagnostic results on clinical decisions and patient outcomes. Readers are referred to Jaeschke et al. (10, 11) and Deeks (12) for guidance on how to evaluate and interpret articles about diagnostic tests up to this point in the hierarchy which is typically the main focus of evidence-based medicine as it relates to diagnosis.

Thus far, the evidence is necessary but not sufficient for informing resource allocation and health policy. The higher reaches of the evidence pyramid (level 6) are the focus of this chapter, where the cumulative evidence for a test in relation to technical performance, clinical utility, and health outcomes provides the foundation. The cost consequences associated with a test are introduced, where definition of cost is broad and includes not only the "up-front" cost of the test but also the "downstream" costs of treatments prescribed (or avoided) and other cost sequalae of disease that are attributable to the decision to test. The comparative evidence of cost in relation to population health benefit is the metric of value that is useful for those making resource allocation decisions in health policy. The challenges of gathering this evidence in a valid, reliable, and timely way are the focus of this chapter.

OVERVIEW OF ECONOMIC EVALUATION

Economic evaluation in healthcare is a set of formal, quantitative methods used to compare two or more healthcare interventions with respect to their resource use and expected outcomes (13, 14). A full economic evaluation requires the *identification*, *measurement*, and *valuation* of both the clinical benefits of a new intervention and the associated costs. Consideration of both costs and effects enables the estimation of efficiency in order to broaden the evidence base to be more relevant to policymakers responsible for optimizing the use of scarce resources.

How does economic evaluation fit within the context of evidence-based medicine? Evidence-based medicine is the conscientious, explicit, and judicious use of current best evidence in making decisions about the care of individual patients (15). Some have been critical of evidence-based medicine for not including cost considerations in documenting evidence on interventions (16, 17), despite the fact that Cochrane's work discusses costs and efficiency (18). More recently, the Economics Methods Group within the Cochrane Collaboration is developing and encouraging the inclusion of cost considerations as part of the evidence base. Economic evaluation builds on this evidence base by broadening the perspective to include (19, 20):

- consideration of the resource consequences of alternative interventions, and
- methods for valuing health outcomes in a single metric such as quality-adjusted life years or net social benefit.

Approaches to Economic Evaluation

There are three main approaches in a full health economic evaluation; cost–benefit analysis (CBA), cost–effectiveness analysis (CEA) and cost–utility analysis (CUA) (Table 1). All three approaches require that both cost and benefits be measured. They differ in how effectiveness is measured and whether or not effectiveness is valued in terms of money.

In the past few decades, the number of economic evaluations published in the medical literature has grown rapidly (21). Of the 3200 eligible articles identified in a review of CBA and CEA articles from 1979 through 1990, approximately 1000 were of diagnostic interventions (22). In a separate review focused on published economic evaluations of diagnostic tests (which included both laboratory and imaging technologies), CEA was the type of

Table 1
Approaches to economic evaluation [adapted from (20)]

Approach	Costs	Benefits
Cost–benefit analysis (CBA)	Money (e.g., dollars)	Money (e.g., dollars)
Cost–effectiveness analysis (CEA)	Money (e.g., dollars)	Natural units (e.g., life years)
Cost–utility analysis (CUA)	Money (e.g., dollars)	Combine quantity and quality of life (e.g., QALYs)

economic evaluation most frequently used. None of the 134 abstracts were CBA, 47% were CEA, and 7% were CUA analyses (23).

Cost–Benefit Analysis (CBA)

In a CBA, consequences are valued in monetary units, which may be any kind of currency (e.g., U.S. dollars or Euros). The goal of cost–benefit analysis is to determine whether the benefits of an intervention exceed its costs. Cost-benefit analysis is suited to answering the question "Is the intervention worthwhile?" One of the challenges of CBA is that health outcomes must be valued by assigning a dollar amount to a year of life. Although this is routine practice in the transportation and environmental sectors, in healthcare the term "cost–benefit" analysis is often used inappropriately (24) and has not been widely applied. Valuation of health benefits is usually achieved by using either the human capital approach or the willingness-to-pay approach. In the human capital approach, the value of an intervention is based on the impact on a person's productivity and the value of earnings based on wage rates. Willingness-to-pay (WTP) approaches use survey methods to present a hypothetical scenario about an intervention (25). Respondents are asked to state the maximum amount they are willing to pay for the intervention. For example, Raab et al. (26) used a payment card to elicit WTP for a new Pap test using liquid-based cytology technology from a group of 175 women (*see* box on next page). If it were assumed that the new test reduced the risk of dying of cervical cancer from 1 in 37,000 to 1 in 50,000, the mean amount they were willing to pay was $237.

Cost–Effectiveness Analysis (CEA)

In contrast to CBA, CEA and CUA are aimed at answering the question "Given a fixed budget, what is the most efficient way (maximize effective-

---

Willingness to Pay for New Papanicolaou Test Technologies

Scenario
- Assume that your risk of dying of cervical cancer is the same as the average risk for a woman living in Pennsylvania and screened regularly (1 in 37,000).
- By having the new Pap test, the risk of dying of cervical cancer is reduced from 1 in 37,000 to 1 in 50,000.

Question
What is your willingness to pay out-of-pocket for the new Pap test?

Choices
$0, $100, $200, $300, $400, $500, $600, $700, $800, $900, $1000

Responses
- 175 female respondents with mean age of 39 years
- Mean WTP of $237

Adapted from (27).

---

ness) to spend it?" In CEA, effects are measured in one single metric that is a natural unit. Cost effectiveness could be measured in cases of disease averted, change in a physiologic measure such as blood pressure, or change in bone density. For example, a study to evaluate alternative management strategies for patients with suspected peptic ulcer disease used costs per ulcer cured and cost per patient treated as the measures of outcome (27). Two immediate endoscopy and three noninvasive diagnostic and treatment strategies, including serologic testing for *Helicobacter pylori*, were evaluated. On the basis of both outcome measurements, serologic testing was attractive at a cost per ulcer cured of $4541 and a cost per patient treated of $894.

The preferred metric by health economists is one that can be used to compare across diagnostic tests for different diseases. For example, life years or survival is a long-term, downstream measure of outcome that can be used to compare a new liquid-based cytology test for cervical cancer screening (28) and fecal occult blood testing for colorectal cancer (CRC) screening (29). The incremental cost per life year saved of using Papnet technology instead of Autopap technology for cervical cancer rescreening was approximately $147,000 with triennial screening (28). Because the outcome measure metric is cost per life year saved, the cost effectiveness of cervical cancer screening can be compared directly to the cost effectiveness of CRC screening at $92,900 per life year saved for annual rehydrated fecal occult blood testing plus sigmoidoscopy versus unrehydrated fecal occult blood testing plus sigmoidoscopy (29) (Table 2).

Table 2
Cost effectiveness of methods to enhance the sensitivity of Papanicolaou testing for cervical cancer compared to fecal occult blood screening for colorectal cancer [adapted from (28) and (29)]

	Triennial Pap smear	
	Lifetime costs per woman screened, $	Additional days of life per woman screened
With AutoPap-assisted rescreen	$657	25.89
With Papnet-assisted rescreen	$700	26.00
Difference between Papnet and AutoPap	$700 − 657 = $43	~0.11 days
Incremental cost effectiveness	$43/0.11 days = $146,783 per life year saved	

	CRC screening strategy	
	Lifetime costs per person screened, $	Life expectancy, years
UFOBT + SIG every 5 years	$2034	17.4066
RFOBT + SIG every 5 years	$2448	17.4110
Difference between UFOBT and RFOBT strategy	$410	~0.0044
Incremental cost effectiveness	$410/0.0044 = $92,900 per life year saved	

UFOBT, unrehydrated fecal occult blood test; SIG, sigmoidoscopy; RFOBT, rehydrated fecal occult blood test.

Cost–Utility Analysis (CUA)

In CUA, an attempt is made to consider the *quality* of the health outcome in addition to the *quantity* of the health outcome. So, years of life in states less than full health are converted to healthy years based on health state preference values. The result is commonly expressed as *quality-adjusted-life-years (QALYs)*, but other metrics have also been used (30–32). There are a variety of methods that can be used to determine the value assigned to a given health state (33). The three most widely used direct preference-based methods (standard gamble, time-trade off, and visual analogue scale) yield a single score scaled from 0 to 1, representing the worst and best states of health, respectively (14, 20, 34). A number of multiattribute health status classification systems such as Quality of Well Being (35, 36) Health Utilities Index (37–39) and EuroQol (40) have also been developed to avoid the need to measure preferences directly (20). These only require relatively brief surveys to be completed, and scoring formulas are applied to convert the results into utility values.

An example of a cost–utility analysis is the paper published by the Centers for Disease Control Diabetes Cost-Effectiveness Study Group which examined the lifetime costs and benefits of opportunistic screening for diabetes compared with current clinical practice (41). The screening test was performed during a routine physician visit using a fasting plasma glucose test followed by a confirmatory oral glucose tolerance test for those who tested positive. The primary outcome measures included life years saved and QALYs. QALYs were calculated by assigning each year of life without major complications a utility value of 1.0, and major complications a value less than 1 (0.69 for blindness, 0.61 for end-stage renal disease, and 0.8 for lower extremity amputation). Adjustment for quality of life for these complications results in a total 20.51 QALYs compared to 21.11 "unadjusted" life years gained with diabetic screening in a 25–34-year-old cohort (Table 3). Adjustment for quality of life impacts the cost–effectiveness ratio considerably—the cost per QALY is approximately one-third that of the cost per life year estimate. This reflects the fact that in addition to the extension of life achieved through screening for diabetes, there is an additional gain in the quality of those years, thus making the benefit of screening more attractive.

Table 3
Cost effectiveness of screening for Type 2 diabetes [adapted from (41)]

Cohort age 25–34 years	Lifetime costs per person screened	Benefits, life years	Benefits, QALYs
Without screening	$97,360	20.99	20.16
With screening	$102,018	21.11	20.51
Incremental difference	$4658	~0.13	~0.35
Incremental cost effectiveness		$35,768 per life year	$13,376 per QALY

Calculation of Cost–Effectiveness Ratio (ICER)

The underlying calculation of an ICER is the same across all economic evaluation approaches (20). The basic equation is:

$$ICER = \frac{costs_{\text{intervention A}} - costs_{\text{intervention B}}}{effects_{\text{intervention A}} - effects_{\text{intervention B}}}$$

The critical point is that two (or more) alternatives are compared as the *difference in costs* between alternatives divided by the *difference in effects* between alternatives.

ELEMENTS OF A HIGH-QUALITY ECONOMIC EVALUATION

Now that the basic approaches to economic evaluation (CBA, CEA, and CUA) have been reviewed, the key elements common to all economic evaluations are identified and methodological features that should be incorporated into high-quality economic studies are discussed. Although there is no definite consensus on a single best approach to economic evaluation, some basic criteria have been repeatedly identified as important considerations to assess the methodological quality of a published economic study, or to guide users in designing and conducting a high-quality study (42, 43).

Using the well-known 10-point criteria list on methodological quality published by Drummond et al. (20) (Table 4), fecal occult blood tests (FOBT) in screening for CRC will be discussed as an example using the study by Frazier et al. (29). CRC is a leading cause of cancer-related mortality. It is associated with approximately 60,000 deaths per year in the United States and is second only to mortality from cancer of the lung and bronchus (44, 45). Clearly, the resource implications for managing and treating patients with CRC are significant. Screening for CRC makes it possible to identify CRC early, when precursor lesions can be detected and removed and screening for CRC can ultimately reduce mortality (46). However, the only strategy for which effectiveness has been established through randomized controlled trials is FOBT, a laboratory test that is used to detect blood in the stool. Alternative technologies for CRC screening currently available for screening the general population include sigmoidoscopy (SIG), double-contrast barium enema (DCBE), and colonoscopy (COL) (47). These tests vary considerably in many aspects—preparation, procedures, performance, complications, frequency, and cost.

Criteria 1: Was a well-defined economic question specified, examining both costs and outcomes of the intervention in the context of alternatives, with a clearly defined target population, viewpoint, and time horizon?

Table 4
Criteria list for the assessment of methodological quality of economic evaluations of diagnostic testing [Adapted from (20)]

---

1. Was a well-defined economic question specified, examining both costs and outcomes of the intervention in the context of alternatives, with a clearly defined target population, viewpoint, and time horizon?
2. Was a comprehensive description of the competing alternatives provided?
3. Was the effectiveness of the intervention established?
4. Were all the important and relevant costs and consequences for each alternative identified?
5. Were the costs and consequences measured accurately in appropriate physical units?
6. Were costs and consequences valued credibly and appropriately for the type of analysis selected?
7. Were costs and consequences adjusted for differential timing?
8. Was an incremental analysis of costs and consequences of alternative interventions performed?
9. Was allowance made for uncertainty in the estimates of costs and consequences using sensitivity analysis?
10. Did the presentation and discussion of study results address all issues of concern to users?

A well-defined economic question should be specified in a manner that considers both costs and outcomes. A question such as "Is FOBT more costly than COL for CRC screening?" is not an economic efficiency question because it does not include a measure of outcome. Similarly, the question "Is CRC screening using FOBT worth it?" is not sufficient because it does not specify the alternative for comparison. The analysis by Frazier et al. (29) asks the question "What are the consequences, costs, and cost effectiveness of alternative strategies for CRC screening in average-risk individuals?" The study question posed by the investigators of this study considers both costs and outcomes of CRC screening and meets the criteria for a full economic evaluation.

The strategies to be compared and their measures of effectiveness should be stated. The analysis (29) compared 22 different CRC screening strategies, including those specifically recommended by expert panels, and the option of no screening. The measure of effectiveness was life expectancy associated with each of the alternative strategies.

The target population of interest should be described so that the reviewer can judge the context in which the results are valid. In Frazier et al. (29), the target population of "average risk individuals" is further defined as persons representative of the 50-year-old U.S. population based on sex and race.

Investigators could evaluate a diagnostic test from a number of possible viewpoints, and the approach taken should be clearly stated and justified. Possible viewpoints include the patient, the healthcare institution (hospital or health maintenance organization), third-party payer (government or insurance company), or society at large. The most appropriate viewpoint will depend on the specific question being asked, and the perspective of the evaluation may be important in terms of the decisions that can be made. This is especially important for the evaluation of diagnostic tests because the benefit is almost always experienced outside of the laboratory, but the testing costs are borne by the laboratory.

For example, consider the use of cardiac troponin I for risk stratification of patients with chest pain to improve the early identification of patients more likely to progress to more serious cardiac disease. From the viewpoint of the laboratory, adding another test can increase laboratory costs significantly without providing any benefit to the laboratory. Anderson et al. (48) reported an increase of $50 per patient with the implementation of cardiac troponin I testing. The director of the laboratory may not view this to be a good investment if the laboratory is judged solely on the basis of managing within a fixed budget allocation. However, if the viewpoint is broadened to the hospital, then the chief executive officer could very well decide to implement testing with cardiac troponin I because hospital and critical care unit length of stay was reduced significantly and total hospital costs were decreased. The decision to implement rapid, aggressive examination of high-risk patients focused the use of resources to ultimately provide better patient care and lower overall costs to the institution. From an even broader social perspective, appropriate use of the cardiac troponin I laboratory assay increases productivity for low-risk patients who return home sooner and miss less time away from work.

Because economic evaluation is most often directed at informing policy for the purpose of allocating healthcare resources, the broader societal viewpoint is generally advocated by health economists. An economic evaluation done from the societal viewpoint should include nonmedical costs (e.g., patient's time spent in seeking and receiving care and out-of-pocket expenses for travel to receive care) and productivity changes (time off work required to receive care) resulting from the intervention. In the case of CRC screening, this would include time lost from work because of screening tests, subsequent diagnostic follow-up, and treatment if cancer is diagnosed. The article by Frazier et al. (29) states that the study was undertaken from a societal perspective; however, it does not appear that nonmedical or productivity costs are included in the evaluation. The authors do not provide the reasons for excluding these costs.

The time horizon for the study should extend far enough to capture major economic and health outcomes whether they are intended or not. This would include the consequences of additional diagnostic procedures performed as a result of a positive FOBT screening test result, and the possible complications such as perforation of the bowel from a follow-up COL. The analysis by Frazier et al. (29) started at the age of 50 years and assumed that screening or surveillance continued until 85 years of age.

Criteria 2: Was a comprehensive description of the competing alternatives provided?

The competing alternatives to be considered in the analysis should be carefully selected to represent currently available options to estimate the opportunity cost associated with alternative strategies. As already pointed out, cost–effectiveness analysis requires that a comparison be made in the context of (at least) one other alternative. Since an intervention can only be cost effective relative to the specified alternatives, the choice of these alternatives is critical. The comparator is usually the most widely used alternative.

In the evaluation of CRC screening (29), 22 different CRC screening strategies were compared. Analyses of CRC screening published previously have focused on a much smaller number of alternatives and failed to consider all plausible options. Frazier et al. (29) included each of the four main CRC screening technologies (FOBT, SIG, DCBE, COL) in various combinations of frequency (e.g., annual FOBT versus SIG every 5 years versus COL every 10 years), formulation (e.g., rehydrated versus unrehydrated FOBT) and follow-up testing (e.g., FOBT followed by SIG followed by COL if a high-risk polyp is found). The comparator was no screening for CRC. These screening strategies were selected because they included those currently recommended by expert panels, addressed the debate about rehydration with FOBT, and considered alternative approaches to follow-up COL.

Criteria 3: Was the effectiveness of the intervention established?

Before an economic evaluation can be undertaken, evidence of the effectiveness of the intervention is required. An intervention that is not effective cannot be cost effective.

The data to establish effectiveness may come from a variety of sources, including a single randomized controlled trial, a prospective observational study, a retrospective database analysis, or a systematic overview of several studies. It is important to recognize that the design of the study affects the internal validity of the study and therefore, the amount of bias in the results (49, 50). The authors should clearly state what type of data was used as a source of estimating effectiveness. If the evaluation is based on a single study, then details of the design and results of the study should be provided. If the evaluation is based on an overview of a number of studies, then details of how the studies were identified and how the results were synthesized should be provided.

The gold standard for assessing efficacy is the randomized controlled trial because it has the greatest internal validity. By randomizing patients to alternative intervention strategies, differences in outcomes can be attributed to the difference in the strategy rather than other factors. Randomized controlled trials of diagnostic strategies are less common than for treatments. FOBT is the only CRC screening strategy for which efficacy has been established through randomized controlled trials (51–53). Other screening strategies have been evaluated through prospective cohort studies.

However, economic evaluation aims to measure effectiveness—how well the intervention performs under real-world conditions—as opposed to efficacy (54). Consequently, it is ideal if data for an economic evaluation were available from a pragmatic trial, which is usually more generalizable. In a pragmatic trial, subjects are still randomized to alternative treatment groups, but the study protocol does not require double blinding, and the protocol attempts to mimic actual practice as closely as possible (55). If effectiveness data from such well-controlled trials are not available, or relevant economic endpoints have not been measured, or the outcomes do not extend over a sufficiently long enough time horizon, it is often necessary to synthesize data from multiple alternative sources or adapt the data by modeling.

Frazier et al. (29) used a variety of sources to estimate the effectiveness of each CRC screening strategy within the context of a decision analysis model. The final measure of effectiveness estimated was life-years gained. Intermediate measures of diagnostic accuracy (sensitivity for polyps, sensitivity for cancer, and specificity) came from randomized control trial data, prospective studies, and review papers. For example, estimates of 10% sensitivity for polyps, 33% sensitivity for cancer, and 97% specificity for unrehydrated FOBT came from two review papers of these performance characteristics for FOBT that were based on the randomized controlled trial data. These FOBT test performance estimates were combined with autopsy studies and epidemiological data to estimate the age- and sex-specific prevalence of polyps, subsequent incidence among those polyp free at 50 years, and the probability of polyp transformation into cancer. The test performance estimates for SIG and COL were based on a blinded prospective trial.

Criteria 4: *Were all the important and relevant costs and consequences for each alternative identified?*

Although it may not be necessary to include every possible cost and consequence of an intervention, the important and relevant ones should be identified, consistent with the specified viewpoint of the analysis. Cost resource categories may include:

- the healthcare resources consumed (e.g., time of health professionals, medication costs, use of medical equipment and services, and associated capital and overhead costs),
- patient and family resources (e.g., out-of-pocket expenses and the value of their time required for receiving treatment), and
- resources consumed in other sectors (e.g., home care visits and social worker counseling).

The costs included in this analysis (29) were limited to screening test costs and costs associated with CRC treatment. Cancer care often involves significant time for the patient and family, and these costs could be important in the evaluation.

The consequences of an intervention include primarily changes in health state including physical, social, and emotional well-being. Special issues arise in the case of diagnostics tests because of the possible detrimental impact of incorrect diagnoses (false-positive and false-negative tests) (56, 57). Studies that have attempted to quantify these effects have shown that these effects are real and measurable and can influence estimates of cost effectiveness. A separate issue has to do with the value of diagnostic information. Mixed results have been reported about the importance of diagnostic information in health economic evaluation. Hirth et al. (58) reported that the value of diagnostic certainty for peptic ulcer disease was small and insufficient to change cost–effectiveness estimates. However, Raab (59) reported that a patient's willingness to wait for definitive knowledge about the presence of lung cancer could result in large changes in cost–effectiveness estimates. These issues should be explored in future research.

In the Frazier et al. (29) study, the primary outcome was an increase in life expectancy from the reduction in CRC mortality associated with screening. No other outcomes were reported, although adjustment for quality of life could be important because of the poor quality of life associated with CRC.

Criteria 5: Were the costs and consequences measured accurately in appropriate physical units?

Once the important costs and consequences have been identified, they should be measured in appropriate units. Resource use should be presented separately from costs. Examples of resource use measures include total hospital stays in days, number of clinic visits, and the amount and prescription regimen for medications. Costs are measured in dollars (or the appropriate currency) and should be expressed in a constant year (e.g., 2003 dollars), after adjusting by the Medical Care component of the Consumer Price Index as necessary.

In the Frazier et al. (29) study, costs were obtained from a cost study from a large health maintenance organization. Costs included screening test costs, the actual costs of medical personnel and supplies to provide the services, and overhead costs such as administration charting and automated information systems. Individual test costs and lifetime costs of treatment were reported, but the authors failed to provide separate information on resource use. All costs were adjusted and reported in 1998 dollars using the Medical Care component of the Consumer Price Index.

Once the outcomes have been identified, appropriate measurement of the effects should be straightforward. For diagnostic tests, the measure of benefit is commonly an intermediate endpoint rather than a final outcome. Measuring benefits in life years is especially challenging for screening and diagnostic tests because of the complexity of the diagnostic process and the uncertainty about the relationship between diagnosis and outcomes of care (60, 61). For example, in evaluating the effect of adding an automated cardiac troponin I assay to the existing cardiac panel, Anderson et al. (48) measured differences in hospital and cardiac care unit length of stay, time to cardiac catheterization, and hospital and laboratory costs between a control group and a test group. They found a statistically and clinically significant shorter length of stay for the group whose diagnostic cardiac marker testing included cardiac troponin I. However, this benefit was not translated into benefits beyond the hospital admission for these patients.

In the evaluation of CRC screening, measures of effectiveness might focus on the number of polyps detected or number of cases of CRC detected. The study by Frazier et al. (29) was a CEA that measured years of life gained based on the reduction in CRC mortality from screening.

Some examples of economic outcomes for diagnostic tests include:

- Reduced number of clinic visits
- Reduced use of prescription medications
- Reduced length of stay in hospital
- Reduced use of additional inappropriate tests
- Reduced number of hospital readmissions
- Reduced number of emergency visits
- Increased productivity from earlier return to home and work
- Increased life expectancy
- Increased quality-adjusted life expectancy

Criteria 6: Were costs and consequences valued credibly and appropriately for the type of analysis selected?

Costs are normally valued in units of local currency meant to reflect the worth of the resources used and are typically based on the current price for those resources. It is possible to value each resource (hospital days, professional time, treatments), but this approach is very costly. Cost estimates are usually available from institutional accounting systems, fee schedules are typically used to estimate the cost of health professionals, and wholesale prices of medications are quoted as reasonable reflections of cost. In determining whether or not costs were valued credibly, the reader should be cautious of per diem estimates and billed charges. For example, hospital per diem estimates are likely to overestimate or underestimate the actual cost for a particular stay. Likewise, billed charges do not represent costs (62). If charges are the only estimates available, then it is recommended that an adjustment be made using an estimate of the cost-to-charge ratio, or the authors should clearly state how these estimates may influence the results.

In the Frazier et al. (29) study, costs of CRC treatment by stage and time period (initial, continuing, and terminal care) were obtained from a cost study from a large health maintenance organization. No specific details are provided about this costing study, but it would appear that these estimates should be credible and are neither overall per diem estimates nor charges. No attempt was made to adjust for quality of life or value healthcare benefits in money terms in this study.

Criteria 7: Were costs and consequences adjusted for differential timing?

The time horizon for the study should extend far enough to capture major economic and health outcomes of the alternatives. Particularly when such a long-term time horizon is involved, the results of the study should be adjusted for differences in the timing of costs and consequences. The basis for discounting is that people generally prefer to receive benefits now and delay incurring costs. Discounting allows for this by giving less weight to costs and benefits that occur in the future. There is some controversy in the literature over the rate to use for discounting and whether or not both costs and benefits should be discounted (63). The most common rates used are 3 and 5%, as recommended in various guidance documents (1, 14, 20, 64). Some studies report results discounted at 0, 3, and 5% for comparison. The main point is that authors should report the method used. Given the extended time horizon in the Frazier et al. (29) study, both costs and benefits are appropriately discounted at 3% per year.

Criteria 8: Was an incremental analysis of costs and consequences of alternatives performed?

As is evident from the basic equation used in economic evaluation, the measure of interest is the additional costs of an intervention compared with its additional effects—the incremental cost–effectiveness ratio (ICER). For example, consider two of the CRC screening strategies evaluated in the

Frazier et al. (29) study—no screening and SIG at age 55 years. The measure of effectiveness was the gain in life expectancy and costs were measured as the lifetime cost in U.S. dollars. The ICER is calculated as:

ICER gained

$$= \frac{\text{cost}_{sig} - \text{cost}_{no\ screen}}{\text{life years}_{sig} - \text{life years}_{no\ screen}} = \frac{\$1070 - \$1052}{17.3632 - 17.3481} = \$1200 \text{ per life year saved}$$

Note that it would be incorrect to compare the ratio of costs to outcomes for each of the two alternatives (i.e., $\$1070/17.3632 = \$61.62$ for no screening and $\$1052/17.3481 = \$60.64$ for SIG). This would be the average cost–effectiveness ratio, and is not relevant for economic evaluation.

The results of an economic evaluation can be categorized into one of three groups, depending on whether the new intervention is more costly than, less costly than, or of equivalent cost to the alternative and whether it is more effective, less effective, or equally effective. This can be illustrated graphically on a four-quadrant diagram (Figure 2) referred to as the cost–effectiveness plane (13, 20, 65).

What are the possibilities?

- Accept new intervention: Under the assumption that all other things are equal, any new intervention that is more effective but costs the same or less than the alternative should be adopted. In addition, if the effectiveness is the same but costs are less, the new intervention should be adopted. This result falls in quadrant D (southeast) of Figure 2.
- Reject new intervention: Under the assumption that all other things are equal, any new intervention that is less effective, but costs the same or more than the alternative should be rejected. In addition, if the effectiveness is the same, but costs more, the new intervention should be rejected. This result falls in quadrant B (northwest) of the cost–effectiveness plane (Figure 2).
- Consider other reasons: In quadrants A and C, there is no obvious decision. Other reasons why it might be beneficial to adopt the new technology need to be considered. If a new intervention is less effective and less costly than the alternative, then it must be decided if the loss in effect is acceptable. If the new intervention and the alternative are equally effective and costly, then other reasons why it should or should not be adopted need to be considered. A new intervention that is more effective but also more costly requires a decision about whether or not the added effect is worth the added cost. Most new technologies fall in this category because they are better than older technologies, but they are more expensive to produce.

Most new technologies fall into the category where the technology is more effective, but also more costly (northeast quadrant A). In the Frazier

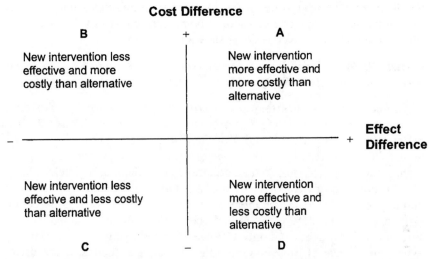

Cost Difference

B | + | **A**

New intervention less effective and more costly than alternative

New intervention more effective and more costly than alternative

Effect **Difference**
−   +

New intervention less effective and less costly than alternative

New intervention more effective and less costly than alternative

C − **D**

Figure 2 The cost–effectiveness plane [adapted from (65)].

In the diagram, the horizontal axis represents the effect difference between the new intervention and the alternative. The vertical axis represents the cost difference between the new intervention and the alternative. The alternative is considered to lie at the intersection of both axes.

If the new intervention lies in quadrant B (northwest) or D (southeast), then the choice between interventions is clear. In quadrant B, the new intervention is both less effective and more costly than the alternative (it is dominated by the alternative). In quadrant D, the new intervention is both more effective and less costly than the alternative (it dominates the alternative). In quadrants A and C, the choice depends on the amount that society is willing to pay for the new technology.

et al. (29) study, seven strategies were identified for which incremental ICERs were calculated ranging from $1200 (SIG once at 55 years) to $92,900 (rehydrated FOBT plus SIG every 5 years) per life year saved. Once these estimates have been derived from a study, the question is then "What is an acceptable price to pay for saving an additional year of life?" The answer to this will depend on external factors or criteria that reflect what a society is willing to pay for this improvement. A threshold of $50,000 per QALY is often quoted as a point of reference for interpreting cost–effectiveness ratios (66). In the United States, this figure refers back to a decision made by the U.S. Congress to approve treatment for end-stage renal dialysis, but there is no empirical basis for it. Investigators have debated the theoretical validity of interpreting cost–effectiveness ratios relative to a fixed threshold (67, 68). In addition, there are practical problems of comparing cost–effectiveness studies that may have used very different methods, data, and assumptions (69).

In analyses where there are multiple alternatives to compare, calculating the incremental cost–effectiveness ratio is more difficult. An illustration of how an incremental analysis should be performed when there are more than two alternatives to consider is shown in Table 5.

Criteria 9: *Was allowance made for uncertainty in the estimates of costs and consequences using sensitivity analysis?*

Some degree of uncertainty is inherent in every economic evaluation. In evaluating CRC screening, examples of uncertain assumptions and estimates include the natural history of CRC, the effectiveness of screening with FOBT, the resource use associated with screening and subsequent management of CRC, uptake and adherence to screening regimens, etc.

Authors should identify the critical assumptions adopted in the analysis and data estimates for which there is uncertainty. A review by Briggs et al. (70) reported that 25% of published economic evaluations failed to consider uncertainty at all, and only 14% were judged to have done it well. To assess the effects of these assumptions and data estimates, a sensitivity analysis should be performed by reworking the analysis under alternative assumptions. The purpose of sensitivity analysis is to examine the robustness of a result over a range of alternative values for uncertain parameters (20, 71). If large variations in the assumptions or data estimates do not produce significant changes in the results, then the confidence level about the results is increased.

Different approaches to sensitivity analysis include one-way or multiple-way sensitivity analysis (varying one or more estimates). Best-case and worst-case scenarios can also be presented where all the critical estimates are simultaneously varied to their most optimistic and most pessimistic values. Frazier et al. (29) performed extensive sensitivity analyses, but this was limited to one-way analyses. They found a significant amount of variability in the results. The ICER of rehydrated FOBT plus SIG every 5 years compared to unrehydrated FOBT plus SIG every 5 years varied from being more costly (but of equal effectiveness) to $248,000 per life year saved. The base case estimate was $92,900 per life year saved.

The simpler approaches to sensitivity analysis listed are limited, and probabilistic sensitivity analyses by Monte Carlo simulation methods are growing in popularity (72, 73). For economic analyses of trial data where individual level values for costs and effects are available (stochastic data with a mean and variance), it is now expected that statistical significance be tested. A point estimate for the ICER should be provided with confidence intervals, along with details of the statistical tests performed. Readers are referred to other sources for a detailed discussion of alternative methods for dealing with uncertainty and guidelines on reporting sensitivity analysis (71, 74–78).

Criteria 10: *Did the presentation and discussion of study results address all issues of concern to users?*

Table 5
Calculation of incremental cost–effectiveness ratio (ICER) with more than two strategies [adapted from (29)]

CRC screening strategy	Cost per person	Life expectancy	ICER	
Other screening strategies				
1. UFOBT + SIG every 10 years	$1810	17.4022	$21,200[a]	
2. RFOBT	$1986	17.3991	...	More costly, less effective than strategy 1. Eliminated by dominance as per step 1.
3. UFOBT + SIG every 5 years	$2034	17.4066	$51,200	ICER compared to strategy 2 = ($2034 − $1986)/ (17.4066 − 17.3991).
4. RFOBT + SIG every 10 years	$2226	17.4078	...	More costly, more effective than strategy 3, but ICER is greater than strategy 5. Eliminated by extended dominance as per step 4.
5. RFOBT + SIG every 5 years	$2448	17.4110	$92,900	ICER compared to strategy 4 = ($2448 − $2226)/ (17.4110 − 17.4078).

[a] This is the ICER for UFOBT + SIG every 10 years compared to the next most efficient alternative (not shown here). UFOBT, unrehydrated fecal occult blood test; RFOBT, rehydrated fecal occult blood test; SIG, sigmoidoscopy.

When more than two strategies are involved, calculation of the correct incremental cost–effectiveness ratio is more complicated. The analysis involves a series of steps to determine the appropriate comparisons to be made. Each alternative should be compared with the next most efficient alternative (20). This approach can be illustrated with a subset of the comparisons from the Frazier et al. (29) study. **Step 1:** Eliminate strategies that are more costly and less effective than an alternative (dominance). **Step 2:** Rank order the strategies by increasing effectiveness. **Step 3:** Calculate the ICER for each strategy compared with the next least expensive strategy. **Step 4:** Eliminate strategies with a lower effectiveness and higher cost–effectiveness ratio than another strategy (extended dominance). **Step 5:** Recalculate the ICER for each strategy compared with the next least expensive strategy.

There are many decisions required in undertaking an economic evaluation. In presenting the study results, the authors should make it clear to the reader what decisions were made and why.

It is important that the results answer all aspects of the initial question defined at the outset. The study by Frazier et al. (29) asked "What are the consequences, costs, and cost effectiveness of alternative strategies for CRC screening in average-risk individuals?" The results addressed this question by evaluating 22 alternative CRC screening strategies. The lifetime cost and life expectancy were reported separately in addition to the calculated ICER.

The conclusions should be consistent with the results. Frazier et al. (29) summarized the results and concluded that screening for CRC significantly reduced CRC mortality at costs comparable to other cancer screening programs. Studies should also include a discussion of the study results compared with those of previously published reports. Frazier et al. (29) compared their results with two other mathematical models of the cost effectiveness of CRC screening, and other cancer screening programs (annual Papanicolaou testing for cervical cancer at $99,000 per life year saved and annual mammography for women ages 55–64 years at $132,000 per life year saved).

Most importantly, the authors should discuss the limitations of their study and their effect on the study conclusions. Frazier et al. (29) discuss several limitations of their analysis. Many of these were related to the uncertainty about the natural history of CRC. Another limitation they identified was the assumption that the test performance of FOBT was the same for initial and repeated tests, which they determined could bias the results toward strategies with FOBT.

SPECIAL CHALLENGES OF ECONOMIC EVALUATION OF DIAGNOSTIC TESTS— A RESEARCH AGENDA

The economic evaluation of diagnostic tests is important, but it does present some particular challenges. The quality of such evaluations could be improved. The complexity of the diagnostic process over the long term further complicates analysis. And finally, the impact of diagnostic information must be considered.

Quality of Economic Evaluations

Although the number of economic evaluations published in the medical literature has grown, from a methodological perspective, economic evaluations of diagnostic technologies do not generally adhere well to the guidelines discussed here for reporting economic evaluations. An analysis of 250 economic evaluations of diagnostic technologies between 1992 and 1997 showed that only about half (134 papers) met two of the basic criteria for an economic evaluation–the first that it must include a comparison of two or more alternatives, and the second that it must consider both costs and outcomes (23). This likely leads to the suboptimal use of information from economic evaluations about diagnostic technologies. If the results of such analyses are to influence decision making, then more consistent adherence to the discussed criteria for high-quality economic evaluation is required in future research.

Complexity of the Diagnostic Process in Long-Term Perspective

Economic evaluation of diagnostic technologies is particularly challenging because of the complexity and hierarchical nature of the diagnostic and subsequent treatment process (60, 61). For example, screening for CRC is a complex series of decisions that begins with the screening test (79). Test performance characteristics such as sensitivity and specificity need to be translated into information about the diagnostic accuracy of the test (8, 10–12, 80). Some patients will be incorrectly diagnosed–either falsely identified as having the disease or falsely identified as not having the disease. Most evaluations of diagnostic tests stop here (81).

However, outcomes also depend on the subsequent treatment, for which there could be many options. The most widely recognized problem of evaluating diagnostic tests is capturing the whole chain of outcomes that arise—the diagnostic test and the treatment intervention are inextricably linked (60). However, the value of achieving the outcome tends to be attributed to the intervention, despite the fact that appropriate treatment can only be accomplished on the basis of correct diagnosis. An example where alternative approaches to delivering care can also affect outcomes is point-of-care testing (82). Self-testing for blood glucose and clinic glycated hemoglobin can improve glycemic control, delay the onset of complications of diabetes, and lead to improved clinical and economic outcomes (83–85). Nonetheless, on the basis of cost per test, point-of-care testing is generally more expensive (86).

For health economics, the consequences of subsequent changes in patient management and treatment decisions are most useful if they are translated into long-term outcomes such as additional years of life or QALYs. Costs need to include all downstream expenses associated with subsequent diagnostic procedures, cancer treatment and patient care, and complications resulting from testing and treatment. Demonstrating the downstream value of diagnostic testing by connecting intermediate endpoints to final patient outcomes and measures of efficiency almost always requires some kind of decision analytic modeling (60, 61, 87). The use of decision modeling to predict long-term clinical and economic outcomes where multiple sources of clinical and cost data are combined is gaining popularity and acceptance (88). Methodological advances to deal with uncertainty in decision modeling where multiple sources of data are required may also encourage the acceptability of modeling to policymakers.

Impact of Diagnostic Information

Diagnostic information has value in addition to the health outcomes that can be routinely captured in an economic evaluation. Test results can generate feelings of distress from the knowledge of disease or feelings of reassurance from the knowledge of being free of disease (57, 89, 90). However, these elements are not captured by conventional outcome measures such as life years or QALYs. QALYs are insensitive to the transient health states experienced during diagnostic procedures and fail to explicitly recognize less tangible outcomes such as the value of information to the consumer (91). Particularly in the context of screening tests, the impact of diagnostic error (false-positive or false-negative results) may be substantial. The detrimental effects of treating those without the disease as a result of a false-positive test result also need to be considered. Economic methods that estimate the effect of a patient's risk-taking and willingness to pay for diagnostic certainty have been applied to diagnostics (58, 59) but have not been widely adopted. This is an another area for further research.

SUMMARY

This chapter has shown how economic evaluation can build on the evidence base to help determine the value of diagnostic laboratory tests in the context of the efficient use of healthcare resources. An overview of the main approaches to economic evaluation was presented and the key elements for assessing the methodological quality of economic evaluations were outlined using the example of fecal occult blood testing to screen for colorectal cancer. Finally, some of the specific methodological challenges and opportunities for research in the economic evaluation of diagnostic tests were highlighted. In summary, the key messages from the chapter include:

- In order to establish the value of a diagnostic test in the context of competing demands for healthcare dollars, there needs to be a shift in the way practitioners think about diagnostic tests. Economic evaluation provides some of the tools needed to achieve this.
- A full economic evaluation requires the *identification, measurement,* and *valuation* of both the clinical benefits of a new intervention and the associated costs. Consideration of both costs and effects enables the estimation of efficiency to broaden the evidence base to be more relevant to policy makers responsible for optimizing the use of scarce resources.
- There are well-accepted criteria for assessing economic evaluations.

These apply equally as well to economic evaluations of diagnostic tests, and studies should be critically reviewed and planned using these criteria as a guide.

- Demonstrating the downstream value of diagnostic testing by connecting intermediate endpoints to final patient outcomes and measures of efficiency almost always requires some kind of decision analytic modeling.
- Economic methods that estimate the effect of a patient's risk-taking and willingness to pay for diagnostic certainty have been applied to diagnostics but have not been widely adopted. This is an area for further research.

REFERENCES

1. Canadian Coordinating Office for Health Technology Assessment. Guidelines for economic evaluation of pharmaceuticals: Canada. Ottawa: CCOHTA, 1994.
2. Taylor R. National Institute for Clinical Excellence (NICE). HTA rhyme and reason? Int J Technol Assess Health Care 2002;18:166–70.
3. National Institute for Clinical Excellence (NICE): symposium on technology assessment. Int J Technol Assess Health Care 2002;18:159–212.
4. Department of Health, Commonwealth of Australia. Guideline for the pharmaceutical industry on preparation of submissions to the Pharmaceutical Benefits Advisory Committee: including submissions involving economic analysis. Woden (ACT), 1990.
5. Smith CS, Hailey D, Drummond M. The role of economic appraisal in health technology assessment: the Australian case. Soc Sci Med 1994;38:1653–62.
6. Drummond MF, O'Brien BJ, Stoddart GL, Torrance GW. Methods for economic evaluation of health care programmes, 2nd ed. Oxford: Oxford University Press, 1997.
7. Fryback DG, Thornbury JR. The efficacy of diagnostic imaging. Med Decis Making 1991;11:88–94.
8. Guyatt GH, Tugwell P, Feeny D, Haynes RB, Drummond M. A framework for clinical evaluation of diagnostic technologies. Can Med Assoc J 1986;134:587–94.
9. Silverstein MD, Boland BJ. Conceptual framework for evaluating laboratory tests: case-finding in ambulatory patients. Clin Chem 1994;40:1621–7.
10. Jaeschke R, Guyatt G, Sackett DL, for the Evidence-Based Medicine Working Group. Users' guides to the medical literature. III. How to use an article about a diagnostic test. A. Are the results of the study valid? J Am Med Assoc 1994;271:389–91.
11. Jaeschke R, Guyatt G, Sackett DL, for the Evidence-Based Medicine Working Group. Users' guides to the medical literature. III. How to use an article about a diagnostic test. B. What are the results and will they help me in caring for my patients? J Am Med Assoc 1994;271:703–7.
12. Deeks JJ. Using evaluations of diagnostic tests: understanding their limitations and making the most of available evidence. Ann Oncol 1999;10:761–8.
13. O'Brien BJ, Heyland D, Richardson WS, Levine M, Drummond MF. Users' guides to the medical literature XIII. How to use an article on economic

analysis of clinical practice. B: What are the results and will they help me in caring for my patients? J Am Med Assoc 1997;277:1802–6.

14. Gold MR, Siegel JE, Russell LB, Weinstein MC. Cost-effectiveness in health and medicine. Oxford: Oxford University Press, 1996.

15. Sackett DL, Rosenberg WMC, Gray JAM, Haynes RB, Richardson WS. Evidence based medicine: what it is and what it isn't. Br Med J 1996;312:71–2.

16. Donaldson C, Mugford M, Vale L. From effectiveness to efficiency: an introduction to evidence-based health economics. In: Donaldson C, Mugford M, Vale L, eds. Evidence-based health economics: from effectiveness to efficiency in systematic review. BMJ Books, 2002:1–9.

17. Maynard A. Evidence-based medicine: an incomplete method for informing treatment choices. Lancet 1997; 349:126–8.

18. Cochrane AL. Effectiveness and efficiency: random reflections on health services. London: Nuffield Provincial Hospitals Trust, 1972.

19. Donaldson C, Mugford M, Vale L. Using systematic reviews in economic evaluation: the basic principles. In: Donaldson C, Mugford M, Vale L, eds. Evidence-based health economics: from effectiveness to efficiency in systematic review. BMJ Books, 2002:10–24.

20. Drummond MF, O'Brien B, Stoddart GL, Torrance GW. Methods for the economic evaluation of health care programs, 2nd ed. Toronto: Oxford University Press, 1997.

21. Elixhauser A, Luce BR, Taylor WR, Reblando J. Health care CBA/CEA: an update in the growth and composition of the literature. Med Care 1993;31(suppl 7):js1–js19.

22. Elixhauser A, Halperin M, Schmier J, Luce BR. Health care CBA and CEA from 1991 to 1996: an updated bibliography. Med Care 1998;36:MS1–9.

23. Severens JL, van der Wilt G-J. Economic evaluation of diagnostic tests: a review of published studies. Int J Technol Assess Health Care 1999;15:480–96.

24. Zarnke KB, Levine MA, O'Brien BJ. Cost-benefit analyses in the health-care literature: don't judge a study by its label. J Clin Epidemiol 1997;50:813–22.

25. Gafni A. Willingness to pay. What's in a name? Pharmacoeconomics 1998; – 14:465–70.

26. Raab SS, Grzybicki DM, Hart AR, Kiely S, Andrew-JaJa C, Scioscia E Jr. Willingness to pay for new Papanicolaou test technologies. Am J Clin Pathol 2002;117:524–33.

27. Fendrick AM, Chernew ME, Hirth RA, Bloom BS. Alternative management strategies for patients with suspected peptic ulcer disease. Ann Intern Med 1995;123:260–8.

28. Brown A, Garber A. Cost-effectiveness of 3 methods to enhance the sensitivity of papanicolaou. J Am Med Assoc 1999;281:347–53.

29. Frazier AL, Colditz GA, Fuchs CS, Kuntz KM. Cost-effectiveness of screening for colorectal cancer in the general population. J Am Med Assoc 2000;284:1954–61.

30. Nease RF. Utility assessment and clinical trials of diagnostic interventions. Acad Radiol 1999;6(suppl 1):S103–S108.

31. Gafni A, Birch S, Mehrez A. Economics, health and health economics: HYEs versus QALYs. J Health Econ 1993;12:325–39.

32. Gafni A. Alternatives to the QALY measurement for economic evaluations. Support Care Cancer 1997;5:105–11.

33. Spilker B. Quality of life and pharmacoeconomics in clinical trials. 2nd ed. Philadelphia: Lippincott-Raven, 1996.

34. Torrance GW. Measurement of health state utilities for economic appraisal: a review. J Health Econ 1986;5:1–30.

35. Kaplan RM, Anderson JP. The general health policy model: an integrated approach. Quality of life and pharmacoeconomics in clinical trials. Philadelphia: Lippincott-Raven, 1996:309–22.

36. Kaplan RM, Anderson JP. A general health policy model: update and applications. Health Serv Res 1988;23:203–35.

37. Feeny D, Furlong W, Boyle M, Torrance GW. Multi-attribute health status classification systems: health utilities index. Pharmacoeconomics 1995;7:490–502.

38. Feeny D, Torrance GW, Labelle R. Integrating economic evaluations and quality of life assessments. Quality of life and pharmacoeconomics in clinical trials. Philadelphia: Lippincott-Raven, 1996:85–95.

39. Torrance GW, Furlong W, Feeny D, Boyle KF. Multi-attribute preference functions: Health utilities index. Pharmacoeconomics 1995;7:503–20.

40. Kind P. The EuroQol instrument: an index of health-related quality of life. Quality of life and pharmacoeconomics in clinical trials. Philadelphia: Lippincott-Raven, 1996: 191–201.

41. CDC Diabetes Cost-Effectiveness Study Group. The cost-effectiveness of screening for type 2 diabetes. J Am Med Assoc 1998;280:1757–63.

42. Ament A, Evers S, Goossens M, De Vet H, Van Tulder M. Criteria list for conducting systematic reviews based on economic evaluation studies—the CHEC project. In: Donaldson C, Mugford M, Vale L, eds. Evidence-based Health Economics: From effectiveness to efficiency in systematic review. BMJ Books, 2002:99–113.

43. Drummond M, Jefferson TO. Guidelines for authors and peer reviewers of economic submissions to the BMJ. Br Med J 1996;313:275–83.

44. Winawer SJ, Fletcher RH, Miller L, Godlee F, Stolar MH, Mulrow CD, et al. Colorectal cancer screening: clinical guidelines and rationale. Gastroenterology 1997;112:594–642.

45. Smith RA, von Eschenback AC, Wender R, Levin B, Byers T, Rothenberger D, et al. American Cancer Society guidelines for the early detection of cancer: update of early detection guidelines for prostate, colorectal, and endometrial cancers. CA Cancer J Clin 2001;51:38–75.

46. Detsky AS. Screening for colon cancer: Can we afford colonoscopy? N Engl J Med 2001;345(8):607–8.

47. Rex DK, Johnson DA, Lieberman DA. Colorectal cancer prevention 2000: screening recommendations of the American College of Gastroenterology. Am J Gastroenterol 2000;95:868–77.

48. Anderson FP, Fritz ML, Kontos MC, McPherson RA, Jesse RL. Cost-effectiveness of cardiac troponin I in a systematic chest pain evaluation protocol: use of cardiac troponin I lowers length of stay for low-risk cardiac patients. Clin Lab Manage Rev 1998;12:63–9.

49. U.S. Preventive Services Task Force. Guide to clinical preventive services. Baltimore, MD: Williams & Wilkins, 1989.

50. Canadian Task Force on Preventative Health Care. Colorectal cancer screening. Can Med Assoc J 2001;165:206–8.

51. Hardcastle JD, Chamberlain JO, Robinson MH, Moss SM, Amar SS, Balfour TW, et al. Randomised controlled trial of faecal-occult-blood screening for colorectal cancer.[Comment]. Lancet 1996;348:1472–7.

52. Kronborg O, Fenger C, Olsen J, Jorgensen OD, Sondergaard O. Randomised study of screening for colorectal cancer with faecal-occult-blood test.[Comment]. Lancet 1996;348:1467–71.

53. Mandel JS, Bond JH, Church TR, Snover DC, Bradley GM, Shuman LM, et al. Reducing mortality from colorectal cancer by screening for fecal occult blood. Minnesota colon cancer control study.[Comment][erratum appears in N Engl J Med 1993;329:672]. N Engl J Med 1993; 328:1365–71.

54. Coyle D, Davies L, Drummond MF. Trials and tribulations. Emerging issues in designing economic evaluations alongside clinical trials. Int J Technol Assess Health Care 1998;14:135–44.

55. Glick HA, Polsky D, Schulman KA. Trial-based economic evaluations: an overview of design and analysis. In: Drummond M, McGuire A, eds. Economic evaluation in health care: merging theory with practice. New York: Oxford University Press, 2001:113–40.

56. Sox HC, Margulies I, Sox CH. Psychologically mediated effects of diagnostic tests. Ann Intern Med 1981;95:680–5.

57. Marshall KG. Prevention. How much harm? How much benefit? 3. Physical, psychological and social harm. Can Med Assoc J 1996;155:169–76.

58. Hirth RA, Bloom B, Chernew M, Fendrick M. Willingness to pay for diagnostic certainty. J Gen Intern Med 1999;14:193–5.

59. Raab SS. The effect of a patient's risk-taking attitude on the cost effectiveness of testing strategies in the evaluation of pulmonary lesions. Chest 1997;111:1583–90.

60. Sassi F, McKee M, Roberts JA. Economic evaluation of diagnostic technology. Methodological challenges and viable solutions. Int J Technol Assess Health Care 1997;13:613–30.

61. Mushlin AI, Ruchlin HS, Callahan MA. Cost effectiveness of diagnostic tests. Lancet 2001;358:1353–5.

62. Finkler SA. The distinction between costs and charges. Ann Intern Med 1982;102–9.

63. Gravelle H, Smith D. Discounting for health effects in cost-benefit and cost-effectiveness analysis. Health Econ 2001;10:587–99.

64. Weinstein MC, Stason WB. Foundations of cost-effectiveness analysis for health and medical practices. N Engl J Med 1977;196:716–21.

65. Black WC. A graphic representation of cost-effectiveness. Med Decis Making 1990;10:212–4.

66. Laupacis A, Feeny D, Detsky AS, Tugwell P. How attractive does a new technology have to be to warrant adoption and utilization? Tentative guidelines for using clinical and economic evaluations. Can Med Assoc J 1992;146:473–81.

67. Johannesson M, Weinstein MC. On the decision rules of cost-effectiveness analysis. J Health Econ 1993;12:459–67.

68. Birch S, Gafni A. Changing the problem to fit the solution: Johannesson and Weinstein's (mis)application of economics to real world problems. J Health Econ 1993;12:469–76.

69. Drummond MF, Torrance GW, Mason J. Cost-effectiveness league tables: more harm than good? Soc Sci Med 1993;37:33–40.

70. Briggs AH, Sculpher MJ. Sensitivity analysis in economic evaluation: a review of published studies. Health Econ 1995;4:355–71.

71. Briggs AH, Sculpher M, Buxton M. Uncertainty in the economic evaluation of health care technologies: the role of sensitivity analysis. Health Econ 1994; 3:95–104.

72. Doubilet P, Begg CB, Weinstein MC, Braun P, McNeil BJ. Probabilistic sensitivity analysis using Monte Carlo simulation. A practical approach. Med Decis Making 1985;5:157–77.

73. Briggs AH, Mooney CZ, Wonderling DE. Constructing confidence intervals around cost-effectiveness ratios: an evaluation of parametric and non-parametric methods using Monte Carlo simulation. Stat Med 1999;18:3245–62.

74. Briggs AH. Handling uncertainty in economic evaluation. Br Med J 1999;319:120.

75. Briggs AH, Wonderling DE, Mooney CZ. Pulling cost-effectiveness analysis up by its bootstraps: a non-parametric approach to confidence interval estimation. Health Econ 1997;6:327–40.

76. O'Brien BJ, Drummond MF, Labelle RJ, Willan A. In search of power and significance: issues in the design and analysis of stochastic cost-effectiveness studies in health care. Med Care 1994;32:150–63.

77. Willan AR, O'Brien BJ. Sample size and power issues in estimating incremental cost-effectiveness ratios from clinical trials data. Health Econ 1999;8:203–11.

78. Chaudhary MA, Stearns SC. Estimating confidence intervals for cost-effectiveness ratios: an example from a randomized trial. Stat Med 1996; 15:1447–58.

79. Lieberman DA. Cost-effectiveness model for colon cancer screening. Gastroenterology 1995;109:1781–90.

80. Greenhalgh T. Papers that report diagnostic or screening tests. Br Med J 1997; 315:540.

81. Raab SS. The cost-effectiveness of immunohistochemistry. Arch Pathol Lab Med 2000;124:1185–91.

82. Price CP. Point of care testing. Br Med J 2001;322:1285–8.

83. Diabetes Control and Complications Trial Research Group. The diabetes control and complications trial—implications for policy and practice. N Engl J Med 1993;329:977–86.

84. UKPDS Group. Intensive blood glucose control with sulphonylureas or insulin compared with conventional treatment and risk of complications in patients with type 2 diabetes (UKPDS 33). Lancet 1998;352:837–53.

85. Grieve R, Beecher RC, Vincent J, Mazurkiewicz J. Near patient testing in diabetes clinics: appraising the costs and outcomes. Health Technol Assess 1999;3:1–74.

86. Dahler-Eriksen BS, Lauritzen T, Lassen J, Lund ED, Brandslund I. Near-patient test for C-reactive protein in general practice: assessment of clinical, organizational, and economic outcomes. Clin Chem 1999;45:478–85.

87. Buxton MJ, Drummond MF, Van Hout BA, Prince RL, Sheldon TA, Szucs T,

et al. Modelling in economic evaluation: an unavoidable fact of life. Health Econ 1997;6:217–27.

88. O'Brien B. Economic evaluation of pharmaceuticals: Frankenstein's monster or vampire of trials? McMaster—CHEPA—Working Paper 95–6, 1995.

89. Dominitz JA, Provenzale D. Patient preferences and quality of life associated with colorectal cancer screening. Am J Gastroenterol 1997;92:2171–8.

90. Mushlin AI, Mooney C, Holloway RG, Detsky AS, Mattson DH, Phellps CE. The cost-effectiveness of magnetic resonance imaging for patients with equivocal neurological symptoms. Int J Technol Assess Health Care 1997;13:21–34.

91. Mushlin AI, Mooney C, Grow V, Phelps CE. The value of diagnostic information to patients with suspected multiple sclerosis. Arch Neurol 1994;51:67–72.

10

From Evidence to Guidelines

David E. Bruns and Wytze P.Oosterhuis

Evidence-based medicine provides important tools to identify and synthesize current best evidence for the care of patients. The conduct of well-designed primary studies and their full and transparent reporting cannot, however, guarantee improved patient care, nor can the preparation and publication of high-quality systematic reviews. An important next step is the application of the findings, a task that increasingly makes use of clinical practice guidelines.

The era of evidence-based medicine has seen an explosive growth in the number of such documents intended to guide clinical practice. A PubMed search in January 2003 on "guidelines AND clinical" returned 22,253 papers. Adding "AND laboratory" to the search returned 1698 papers (~8 % of the total). While not all of these papers are relevant to clinical practice guidelines and laboratory medicine, a full text search of *Clinical Chemistry* for the period 1997–2003 for the word "guideline" found an impressive 542 papers. Of the most-recent 20 papers in the *Clinical Chemistry* search, 19 were concerned with clinical guidelines, reflecting the considerable recent interest in clinical guidelines among workers in laboratory medicine.

Interest in clinical practice guidelines is widespread and includes the public broadly. According to the *New York Times* (January 24, 2003), the largest health maintenance organization, Kaiser Permanente, will publish on its web site guidelines used by its "doctors for treatment of hundreds of diseases." This information will allow patients and the public to assess the treatment they receive. According to the *Times*, consumer advocates predict that Kaiser's action will prompt other managed care companies and medical groups to make similar disclosures. The *Times* quoted Dr. Carolyn Clancy, acting Director of the U.S. Agency for Healthcare Research and Quality, as saying, "The more stakeholders are engaged in evidence-based medicine, the better." According to the article, more that 50,000 people each month gather information from the web site (http://www.guide-line.gov/index.asp) of the National Guidelines Clearinghouse sponsored by her agency. It seems likely that interest has not peaked.

The motivations to develop guidelines can be multiple, and the altruism of the motivations can sometimes be questioned. A central motivation, of course, common to the likely readers of this book, is a healthy desire to bring the fruits of research to the clinic or bedside. A key driver can be the need to address the wide variability among clinicians in the care of patients. Health systems, however, may be viewed as overly motivated to develop guidelines that will decrease costs at the possible expense of best patient care. This motivation could lead to erroneous decisions to not recommend expensive treatments based on the fallacy that "lack of evidence of effectiveness is evidence of lack of effectiveness." A very different sort of concern can surround guidelines produced by clinician groups that may be suspected of having a financial conflict of interest in recommending potentially self-serving options for diagnosing, monitoring, or treating patients. These considerations are worthy of reflection when developing clinical practice guidelines and suggest the need to follow clear and transparent steps in preparing them.

WHAT, EXACTLY, IS A CLINICAL PRACTICE GUIDELINE?

It is important to be clear about the type of guideline considered here. A widely quoted definition comes from a report of the U.S. Institute of Medicine (1):

> Clinical practice guidelines are systematically developed statements to assist practitioner and patient decisions about appropriate health care for specific clinical circumstances.

This definition appears sufficiently broad to include recent guidelines that focus on use of the clinical laboratory. Examples of the latter in the peer-reviewed, open literature include guidelines for the use of the laboratory in screening, diagnosing, and monitoring hepatic injury (2) and guidelines for laboratory testing in diagnosis and management of diabetes (3).

ISSUES ADDRESSED IN LABORATORY-RELATED GUIDELINES

A listing of issues addressed in recent laboratory-related guidelines reads like a list of issues that laboratorians have always worried about:

Imprecision	Patient preparation
Bias	Sample handling
Frequency of testing	Qualifications of operators
Turnaround time	Selection of test methods
Detection limit	Interferences in methods
Tests to be used	Areas needing research
Tests not to be used	Quality control
Decision limits	External quality assurance
Standardization of assay	Timing of repeat testing
Sample-type for testing	Diagnostic algorithms
Where test is done	Conditions with aberrant results
Diagnostic accuracy	

The key ingredient in clinical practice guidelines is that these issues are related to the "specific clinical circumstances" referred to in the definition of clinical guidelines. This is not to say that laboratorians have not thought this way in the past. The new elements in development of clinical guidelines are the tools of evidence-based medicine outlined in preceding chapters and the formalization of the process of developing guidelines.

It may be argued that some topics covered in laboratory-related guidelines (see above box) are outside the scope of evidence-based medicine. As defined in earlier chapters, evidence-based medicine has its focus on the care of the individual patient, whereas many of the guidelines listed are more related to the science and technology of the laboratory. That distinction will not be addressed in detail in this chapter, but rather comments will be offered to help readers who are involved in developing laboratory-related guidelines, even though some topics may be considered outside the scope of evidence-based medicine. As an example, some earlier guidelines contained pronouncements about such things as analytical goals (e.g., for precision) based solely on "expert opinion" (usually from clinicians). As discussed later, in the development of guidelines, evidence should be brought to bear on issues such as goals for analytical precision, even if that evidence does not seem to be of the type usually associated with evidence-based medicine.

CONCEPTS IN THE DEVELOPMENT OF GUIDELINES

Methods for translating evidence into recommendations or guidelines are less well established than methods for synthesizing evidence (4). A seven-step process for developing guidelines has been proposed that consists of forming multidisciplinary chapter or section development teams; developing a conceptual approach to organizing, grouping, selecting, and evaluating the interventions in each chapter or section of the guideline; selecting interventions to be evaluated; searching for and retrieving evidence; assessing the quality of and summarizing the body of evidence of effectiveness; translating the body of evidence of effectiveness into recommendations; considering information on evidence other than effectiveness; and identifying and summarizing research gaps (4). Woolf pointed out that this process "is slow, laborious, and expensive (sometimes costing hundreds of thousands of dollars)" (5). Schemes that are more or less detailed can be found in the references listed in Appendix 1 and Appendix 2. The authors are unaware of strong evidence on whether use of a simple or complex scheme leads to better guidelines. Steps in a relatively straightforward proposed process (6) are listed in the box below and will be discussed in more detail later.

Regardless of the approach taken, it must be recognized that translation of evidence into practice to improve patient care, though that is the only real goal of accumulating and appraising evidence, remains new territory with pitfalls and costs and a need for evidence and new ideas.

Steps in the development of guidelines

Identify and refine the subject area

Convene and run guideline development groups

Use systematic reviews to assess the evidence

Translate evidence into recommendations

Obtain external review

From (6).

WHERE TO FIND GUIDELINES

Published guidelines not only are useful in themselves, but also provide examples that can guide efforts to produce good guidelines for evidence-based laboratory medicine. A few of the many sources of guidelines are listed in the following box (with Internet addresses) and discussed here.

The **Agency for Healthcare Research and Quality** sponsors the National Guidelines Clearinghouse (NGC). It is a treasure house of information and was reviewed favorably in *Clinical Chemistry* (7). Importantly, the

---

Selected Sources of Guidelines

National Guidelines Clearinghouse
http://www.guideline.gov/index.asp

EBM Guidelines of the Finnish Medical Society
http://www.update-software.com/ebmg/

"Current Guidelines" from Website of the Association of Clinical Biochemists
http://www.acb.org.uk/welshaudit/current_guidelines.htm

National Academy of Clinical Biochemistry
http://www.nacb.org/

NGC has explicit criteria for inclusion of guidelines, as stated on their web site:

1. [It] contains systematically developed statements that include recommendations, strategies, or information that assists physicians and/or other health care practitioners and patients make decisions about appropriate health care for specific clinical circumstances.
2. [It] was produced under the auspices of medical specialty associations; relevant professional societies, public or private organizations, government agencies at the Federal, State, or local level; or health care organizations or plans. . .
3. Corroborating documentation can be produced and verified that a systematic literature search and review of existing scientific evidence published in peer reviewed journals was performed during the guideline development. A guideline is not excluded from NGC if corroborating documentation can be produced and verified detailing specific gaps in scientific evidence for some of the guideline's recommendations.
4. The guideline is English language, current, and the most recent version produced. Documented evidence can be produced or verified that the guideline was developed, reviewed, or revised within the last five years.

This list of criteria can serve as a useful reminder for anyone developing a guideline who wishes to have the guideline listed at websites such as this one. The NGC Update Service will provide email notification when new features and guidelines become available at the web site.

The **Finnish Medical Society** offers Evidence Based Medicine Guidelines on CD and the Internet that include "1000 problem-oriented and disease-specific guidelines." This service requires an annual subscription (99 Euros in 2003).

The **Association of Clinical Biochemists** (UK) posts a useful list of guidelines from Wales. The range of these guidelines is shown in the following box.

"Current guidelines" from Welsh Audit posted on web site of the Association of Clinical Biochemists (accessed January 25, 2003)

Urine microalbumin testing in screening for diabetic nephropathy

Standards for screening for Cushing's syndrome

Biochemical investigation of menopausal status and monitoring of HRT

Trace element analyses and monitoring of TPN

The use of automated immunoassay analyzers

Sweat testing

Monitoring glycemic control in patients with diabetes

Biochemical markers of cardiac damage

Performance of the oral glucose tolerance test

Performance of standards for PSA measurement

Standards for the investigation of serum and urine paraproteins

Standards for thyroid function testing strategies

The **National Academy of Clinical Biochemistry** (NACB) posts guidelines developed under its auspices on its web site. These guidelines are extensively disseminated for comment prior to publication, and those published in *Clinical Chemistry* undergo formal peer review. The method of grading the recommendations in the NACB guidelines varies among the guidelines and often is the system used by the professional clinical society that cosponsors the guidelines. The NACB guidelines, published under the headings of "Standards of Laboratory Practice" or (currently) "Laboratory Medicine Practice Guidelines," appear to meet the criteria for inclusion in the National Guidelines Clearinghouse, and, in fact, it is expected that they soon will be included. (A list of all organizations that are involved with the clearinghouse can be seen at the clearinghouse web site.) The NACB web site also includes drafts of guidelines that are under development.

DEVELOPMENT OF A CLINICAL PRACTICE GUIDELINE

A five-step scheme for development of clinical practice guidelines was described by Shekelle et al. (6). It provides a useful framework for addressing key issues in the process. Not all points found in the original article will be addressed here, and responsibility for the comments about the steps is the authors'. Note that other schemes with seven or up to 10 steps address such things as implementation of guidelines and revision of them after use, steps that take place after the development of the guideline and which are considered separately in this chapter.

Step 1: Identify and Refine the Subject Area

Identifying the exact area to be addressed in a guideline is critical. Its importance may be considered to be analogous to and as important as that of the framing of a clinical question to be addressed in a systematic review. The process can be similarly challenging. If the scope is too broad, any hope of success is lost before beginning. If the subject area is not one that needs attention, the guideline will not attract attention. If the subject area lacks any evidence, the guidelines will be based only on expert opinion and will lack the authority and much of the transparency of an evidence-based process.

Guidelines can address diseases or conditions (e.g., diabetes, cancer, atherosclerosis, or coronary artery disease), symptoms (e.g., chest pain), signs (e.g., abnormal bleeding), or procedures, either therapeutic (e.g., coronary artery bypass grafting) or diagnostic (in the broad sense, including tests for screening and monitoring) (e.g., glucose monitoring, newborn screening, or newborn screening by mass spectrometry).

Shekelle et al. (6) pointed out the importance of prioritizing topics. Priorities may reflect the public health importance of a topic, the extent of variation of practice (often a sign of uncertainty), or a perceived need to reduce costs of care.

A very recent NACB guideline addressed laboratory testing of patients with diabetes. Motivations for this guideline included the alarming increase in obesity and type 2 diabetes and the personal and societal burdens of disease. Another NACB guideline addressed laboratory testing in hepatic diseases, a timely topic because of hepatitis C, among other things.

Once a topic has been agreed upon, the refining of the scope of the guidelines is similarly critical. What are the critical issues to be addressed and which are sufficiently peripheral that they can be omitted? Which issues are important clinically? Where do laboratories need guidance? Does the group developing the guidelines have the necessary expertise or can others be brought on board to provide it?

In an ideal world, the process of defining the scope will begin in earnest even before the formation of the group that will develop the guidelines. The process will involve serious discussion among clinicians, patients, laboratory experts, and people likely to use and evaluate the guidelines. In deciding the scope of the guidelines, consideration must be given to the time and resources available. What staff support will be provided to the team? What is the budget for meetings of the team? As noted elsewhere (6), "It is possible to develop guidelines that are both broad in scope and evidence based, but to do so requires considerable time and money, both of which are frequently underestimated by inexperienced developers of clinical practice guidelines."

Example of refining the scope of a guidelines project

In guidelines for testing in diabetes, should lipid testing be addressed? The group planning the NACB guidelines on testing in diabetes faced this question. Some of the potentially relevant considerations are listed in Table 1, and readers are encouraged to think of others.

Testing for lipids is important in diabetes, and one could argue that diabetes might have been considered a disease of lipids rather than of carbohydrates had not practical glucose assays been available before assays for clinically important lipids. As the topic of lipids is a broad one, however, practical considerations included the extent of the resources available for development of guidelines. Similarly, infectious diseases are important in diabetes, but a decision had been made early in the process that microbiological testing was beyond the feasible scope of the guidelines.

The committee charged with developing the NACB guideline on laboratory testing in diabetes decided not to address lipid testing in detail, despite recognition of the importance of the topic. A key concern of the committee was that the guidelines project would become unmanageable if lipid testing were added to diabetes-specific topics that were challenging enough and ranged from glucose meters to glycated hemoglobin and microalbumin testing to genetic and immunological tests.

Did the NACB's committee decide correctly? That is an open question, but it was clear that at least some members of the volunteer committee each devoted 2–3 months' worth of (uncompensated) full-time effort to the project over the 2–3-year period in which the guidelines were developed and promulgated. Enlargement of the scope would have detracted from the effort to focus on key issues and to produce a high-quality document that would win approval by the American Diabetes Association's Clinical Practice Committee. The goal of approval was achieved, but nonetheless the document lacks detailed coverage of an important topic (lipids), and no other guideline has been produced by NACB to address it.

Funding for another new guideline on lipid testing in diabetes may be

Table 1
Pros and cons of including lipid testing in NACB guidelines on laboratory testing in diabetes

Pro: Include lipid testing	Con: Exclude lipid testing
Important area for health	Requires an even larger committee
Active area of research	Would make document too long
Importance may be underappreciated	Would delay completion of guideline
Lipid testing is important in the laboratory	Its importance warrants its own guideline

hard to find. Would a professional association, an insurer (either governmental or private), or a manufacturer or group of manufacturers do so? Depending on the source of funding (if funding could be found), a new guideline may exclude considerations about lipids that are unique to diabetes and might do so for the same kinds of reasons that led to elimination of detailed consideration of lipids in the NACB document on diabetes.

Thus, there are trade-offs in deciding the scope of guidelines. Decisions made early in the process of developing guidelines have important ramifications, some of which can be foreseen if the importance of thinking them through is appreciated, and if people who care devote enough time and thought to planning the scope.

Step 2: Convene and Run Guideline Group

The composition of the guideline development group follows in part from the scope of the proposed guidelines. In laboratory medicine, the team will usually require members from at least two areas, laboratory practice and clinical practice, who are experts on the relevant procedures and conditions. The composition of the guideline development groups has been shown to affect the appraisal of the appropriateness of procedures, with those who perform procedures more likely to favor their use (8). Consideration should be given to including additional individuals who are clearly free of vested interest; such members can bring both credibility and also can be chosen to bring additional expertise in special areas such as statistics, appraising of evidence, and implementation of guidelines and in the processes by which groups reach conclusions. Ideally, staff will be available to the group to retrieve evidence, organize meetings of the group, and coordinate the publication and promulgation of the guidelines (as in audioconferences).

The number of individuals to involve in a guidelines group is an important consideration. It is useful to involve many types of stakeholders, but group sizes larger than about a dozen can be counterproductive if they inhibit an adequate airing of each person's views. A minimum group size of six and a maximum of 12–15 has been recommended (6).

One approach to allowing larger numbers of stakeholders in developing a guideline is to form multiple groups. A steering group may have responsibility for producing the final document, while specialized groups are responsible for assembling and appraising the evidence and making initial recommendations to the steering group. Other scenarios can be envisioned.

Examples of guideline development groups in laboratory medicine

Recently, the NACB perceived a need for two groups of laboratorians to work together in care of people with liver disease and diabetes. In keeping with that real-world aim, the team developing guidelines for liver disease included clinicians from the American Association for the Study of Liver Diseases and the team developing the diabetes guidelines involved the American Diabetes Association. The size of each group (as for other NACB guidelines groups) was within the range recommended. Unfortunately, however, neither guidelines development group included impartial experts in evidence-based medicine or experienced leaders of group processes. Moreover, the groups had no significant staff support for the actual work of developing guidelines. In the diabetes guidelines group (with which one of the authors was involved), each major area of the guideline was the responsibility of a single individual rather than a group, the latter approach having at least the potential to involve more points of view directly in the process.

Based on this example, some suggestions might be considered. In deciding on how to develop the best possible guidelines in laboratory medicine, consideration could well be given to finding funds to support the addition of group members with these additional areas of expertise and to funding for staff support as is common in other groups that develop guidelines. There also appears to be room for the use of several groups (functioning, perhaps, like a steering committee with specialized subcommittees) to develop a guideline, particularly for guidelines on broad topics such as diabetes.

Step 3: Identify and Assess the Evidence

The processes of identifying and assessing evidence have been reviewed earlier in this book. When possible, guidelines can be built on well-performed systematic reviews (ideally more than one) that have been published on the topic. Systematic reviews are necessary when there is expected to be variation between studies, sometimes attributable to effects too small to be measured. Where no systematic reviews exist, the group effectively must undertake to produce one or more as outlined in chapter 7. In performing the review and in appraising published ones, attention must be directed to the category of evidence supporting each conclusion, as this will affect the strength of recommendations made in the guidelines. Thus, for example, if the only available evidence is from a single, small, uncontrolled study, the strength of the resulting recommendation will not be as high as that of a recommendation that follows directly from a meta-analysis of randomized controlled trials.

Step 4. Translate Evidence into a Guideline and Grade the Strength of Recommendations

When the evidence has been gathered and analyzed, the guidelines development group must make recommendations based on the evidence. Here one may be reminded of a cartoon that is well known in some circles: A scientist stands at a blackboard covered with equations that, presumably, develop a suitably complex thesis. Within the string of equations, however, about half way through the argument, a break in the equations contains the words, "Then a miracle occurs." Similarly, in guidelines development, the processes for reaching the best possible recommendations from an expert group are poorly understood. The process may involve balancing of costs and benefits after values are assigned and the strength of evidence is weighed. Conclusive evidence for recommendations is only rarely available. In this situation, authors of guidelines have an ethical responsibility to make very clear the level of evidence that supports each recommendation.

Various schemes are available for grading the level of evidence, and one of them should be adopted and used explicitly. A rather simple one, with a rather typical four levels (A through D), is shown in Table 2. A more elaborate type is shown in Table 3. It includes explicit statement of the type of anticipated benefit from use of a recommended intervention.

The strength of a recommendation does not always map directly to the type of study cited to support it, as recommendations may either follow directly from clinical studies or be extrapolated from the results of the studies. For example, a study supporting use of a drug may have been done very well and thus the evidence may have been graded highly; but if the study was done in adults and the guideline is for children, the strength of the recommendation may be low. Note in Table 2 that the strength of a recommendation that is extrapolated even from a randomized controlled trial (RCT) can be as low as level D.

In the available grading schemes, most or all of which were developed with therapeutic interventions foremost in mind, level A cannot be

Table 2
A scheme for grading of strength of recommendations in clinical guidelines [From (6)]

Level	Characteristics
A	Directly based on meta-analysis of randomized clinical trials (RCTs) or on at least one RCT
B	Directly based on at least one controlled study without randomization or at least one other type of quasi-experimental study or extrapolated from RCTs
C	Directly based on nonexperimental studies or extrapolated from RCTs or nonrandomized studies
D	Directly based on expert reports or opinion or experience of authorities or extrapolated from RCTs, nonrandomized studies or nonexperimental studies

Table 3
Categories of evidence supporting guidelines (A–E) and quality of evidence on which recommendation is based (I–IV) as used by the American Association for the Study of Liver Disease [From (2)]

Category	Explanation
I	Evidence from multiple well-designed randomized controlled clinical trials, each involving a number of patients to be of sufficient statistical power
II	Evidence from at least one large well-designed clinical trial with or without randomization, from cohort or case-controlled analytical studies, or well-designed meta analysis
III	Evidence based on clinical experience, descriptive studies, or reports of expert committees
IV	Not rated
A	Survival benefit
B	Improved diagnosis
C	Improvement in quality of life
D	Relevant pathophysiologic parameters improved
E	Impacts cost of healthcare

achieved without an RCT to support it. As evidence from RCTs is available for only a relatively small number of diagnostic procedures, and then only for restricted groups of patients (or populations), level A evidence is rare in guidelines on use of diagnostic tests.

Even for common tests used in highly prevalent conditions, the strength of evidence for most recommendations achieves only low grades. The recommendations made in the NACB guidelines on laboratory testing in diabetes (3) were graded by the scheme of the American Diabetes Association, a scheme similar to that in Table 2 except that level D is referred to as level E. As shown in Figure 1, the vast majority of the recommendations were graded only as level E (expert opinion) by the authors of the guidelines, and only three were graded as A. A critical reader of the diabetes guidelines might argue that even some of the three recommendations graded as A required extrapolation from the underlying evidence and could just as well have been graded at level B—or even lower. Critical readers will note that the high proportion of recommendations in the NACB document supported only by expert opinion is far from unique or peculiar to that document.

It might be argued that a different grading scheme would be appropriate for guidelines on diagnostic, as opposed to therapeutic, interventions. In fact, it may be argued that the perceived need for RCTs to support strong recommendations is misplaced in the area of diagnostic testing. As pointed

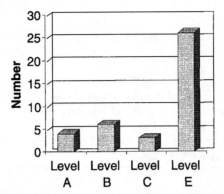

Figure 1 Strength of recommendations in laboratory medicine practice guideline on laboratory testing in diabetes (3).

out by Bossuyt et al. (9), although "the most decisive evidence for judging the effectiveness of diagnostic measures should come from randomised comparisons," randomized comparisons of medical tests are sometimes invalid. Other forms of evidence, particularly observational studies, may need to be given reasonable weight, as these often provide the only available evidence and represent the only evidence likely to become available for some entrenched tests.

Two common issues in laboratory-related guidelines are imprecision and bias (and, now, one should add, total error). Here, the issue is one of goal-setting or "quality specifications" for analytical methods. For such goal-setting efforts, randomized controlled clinical trials (outcomes studies) are difficult to design and are almost never available. Furthermore, it is unlikely that many of them will be available anytime soon, especially for common analytes such as glucose. Is it possible to consider an addition to the grading scheme to allow the use of types of evidence that are not usually considered in evidence-based medicine guidelines?

Fraser and Petersen (10) proposed a hierarchy of evidence (Table 4) that can be used fruitfully for grading certain laboratory-related recommendations. The highest level, related to medical needs, involves consideration of the impact of test performance on medical decision-making in a specific situation. For example, Klee et al. (11) have shown rates of misclassification of cardiac risk as a function of analytical bias of cholesterol assays. Similarly, error rates in insulin dosing can be calculated (12) as a function of imprecision (or bias or both) of glucose measurements (Figure 2). As shown in the figure, increasing imprecision of the glucose assay leads to increasingly frequent errors in the administered dose of insulin. To provide the intended insulin dosage 95% of the time requires that both the bias and the coefficient of variation (CV) of the glucose meter be less than 2%. Although such studies do not demonstrate an effect on patient outcomes, an expert group

Table 4
Hierarchy of criteria for quality specifications [From (10)]

Level	Basis
1 A	Medical decision-making: use of test in specific clinical situations
1 B	Medical decision-making: use of test in medicine generally
2	Guidelines—"experts"
3	Regulators or organizers of external quality assurance schemes
4	Published data on state of the art

can make reasoned recommendations for imprecision based on such data and mathematical modeling when the clinical action follows a well-defined rule.

A randomized controlled trial may add only incrementally to such data. A trial may even be misleading, as outcomes depend on actions by people outside the laboratory. Thus, for example, improving a biochemical test (e.g., creatinine) by eliminating interferences will not necessarily lead immediately to improved outcomes for patients if physicians have not learned that they can rely on the improved assay. In such a scenario, clinical decisions may continue to be made in disregard of the results of the new test when they are not entirely consistent with results of a diagnostically inferior older test (e.g., urea). In this case, patient outcomes would not be improved, and a negative trial would be misinterpreted as providing evidence that the improved assay had no clinical value (whereas the correct interpretation would be that there was a need for improved education).

Level 1B in the scheme for grading evidence for quality specifications (Table 4) refers primarily to the widely used concepts on analytical goals (quality specifications) that are based on within-person and among-person biological variation. These concepts are well established in the laboratory community, but most developers of clinical practice guidelines appear to be woefully unaware of them. Fraser and Petersen (10) spelled out levels of optimum, desirable, and minimum performance for both imprecision and bias based on these concepts. Thus, desirable imprecision produces a CV that is less than half the within-person biological CV, thus ensuring that analytical imprecision plays only a minor role in observed changes in the measured quantity during monitoring. If a test is to be used for monitoring, then use of this type of quality specification is appropriate in guidelines, and an RCT to test it may not even be ethical. Similarly, to allow a common reference interval among methods and laboratories, bias must be less than a reasonable fraction of the biological variation within the population, and Fraser and Petersen have already addressed this in some detail (10).

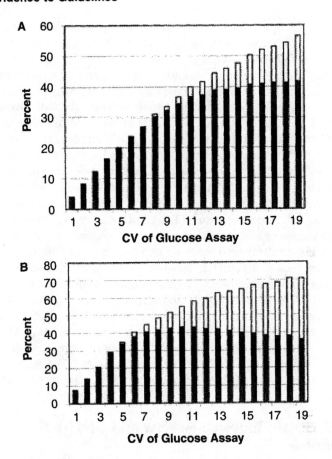

Figure 2 Effect of assay imprecision of glucose assay on administered insulin dose. (Boyd and Bruns, Clin Chem 2001;47:209–14.). Columns show the percentage of cases with insulin dose errors of one (filled columns) or two or more (open columns) categories (or insulin steps). A: Percentages simulated using category (or insulin step) sizes of 50 mg/dL (2.8 mmol/L). B: Percentages simulated using category (or insulin step) sizes of 30 mg/dL (1.67 mmol/L). The bias was set to zero. True glucose concentrations were 150–450 mg/dL (8.3–25 mmol/L). At each CV, 10,000 measurements were simulated to derive the percentages. (Reproduced with permission.)

It is extremely unfortunate that clinical guidelines continue to recommend "CVs" for analytical imprecision (often unspecified as to type, within-run, day-to-day, etc.) that bear no resemblance to the objective criteria related to biological variation (and are not based on medical use of outcomes studies). Data on within-person and among-person biological variation are available for virtually all commonly used tests. The quality specifications relate directly to the ability to use assays for monitoring and ability to use common reference intervals within a population. These may be considered patient-centered objectives if one is willing to stretch the concept. In any event, the world does not need a separate, randomized clinical trial for each analyte to reinvent these fundamental principles. Too often in the past, august groups have declared goals for precision with absolutely no evidence. The time for this is past, and consideration of the levels of evidence of Fraser and Petersen may help when developing laboratory-related guidelines. It is encouraging to see that data on biologic variation are making their way into laboratory-related guidelines, including the recently updated thyroid guidelines from NACB (available on their web site).

It is important to recognize in developing recommendations that the much-maligned "expert opinion" (Table 2, Level D) actually plays a role in almost all recommendations. It is involved, for example, in judgments about extrapolating results from a study on one population to another (e.g., men under 65 and octogenarians), in assessing how representative a small study is of a large population to which a guideline might apply and in making recommendations in the absence of evidence. In all cases, it is recommended that the process for gathering expert opinion be made explicit, and the identity of the experts should be made part of the report. Some NACB guidelines have relied primarily on the working group to prepare all drafts of the guidelines, so that they become the de facto "experts." The drafts, however, undergo review, so that other opinion can and does get incorporated.

Step 5: Obtain External Review and Update the Guidelines

External Review

Shekelle et al. (6) recommended that guidelines be reviewed by at least three types of outside examiners:

- Experts in the clinical content area who would assess completeness of the literature review and the reasonableness of recommendations
- Experts on systematic reviewing and guideline development who would review the process of guideline development
- Potential users of the guidelines

It is not clear that guidelines in laboratory medicine have always included such a structured review.

Guidelines often undergo a formal review process before approval by groups other than the organization primarily responsible for their development. These groups may be other professional societies or government agencies. The processes for such review are not standardized.

Example of reviewing of drafts of guidelines in laboratory medicine

Reviews of drafts of each NACB guideline have been obtained through presentations at (usually several) meetings (including meetings of clinical groups such as the American Thyroid Association), circulation to experts by the working group itself, and postings on the Internet. These comments have led to substantive and valuable revisions of the presented drafts. Groups such as the Clinical Practice Committee of the American Diabetes Association have endorsed several of the guidelines. The documents have also undergone peer review by anonymous reviewers at *Clinical Chemistry*, a process that has, in some cases, lead to further substantive changes (suggesting that the anonymity of a journal's peer-review process sometimes unearths additional views). The journal's peer review, substantive editing, and copyediting have lead to conceptual changes in some cases and have regularly cleared up areas of ambiguity.

Updating of Guidelines

Guidelines constantly become outdated. In a study of clinicians' adherence to a decision-support system for ordering laboratory tests (13), the most frequent type of noncompliance was the addition of tests. Six of the 12 tests most frequently added to the order forms were supported by revisions of guidelines that occurred within 3 years of the time of the ordering of the test. The authors suggested that, in general practice, noncompliance with a guideline is partly caused by practitioners applying new medical insight before it is incorporated in a revision of that guideline.

A recent study assessed the current validity of 17 clinical practice guidelines of the Agency for Healthcare Research and Quality (14). Survival analysis indicated that about half of the guidelines were outdated in 5.8 years (95% confidence interval 5.0–6.6 years). By 3.6 years (CI 2.6–4.6 years), no more that 90% of the conclusions were still valid.

Unfortunately, there is no accepted way to review guidelines and determine when they need to be updated (15). It is probably wise to determine a date for revision as part of the process of developing the guideline. Perhaps better, is to determine a date when the guideline will be reviewed to determine if it needs updating. Two papers (14, 15) address ways in which to review guidelines. The NACB is to be commended for the recently completed revision of the thyroid guidelines.

USING GUIDELINES

Well-developed, evidence-based clinical guidelines have potential for good (and for harm), but their potential depends upon use. Although they can be useful for teaching, their usual intended purpose is implementation. Implementation within a healthcare organization requires "time, enthusiasm and [more] resources" (15). The most important cost is in the time of the experts in the multidisciplinary implementation team that is required. As guidelines have a habit of becoming outdated, the implementation team must have the ability to use tools of evidence-based medicine in finding valid guidelines and in preparing for their implementation. Margolis and Cretin (16) provide guidance on implementation in a book that was reviewed favorably in *Clinical Chemistry*.

SUMMARY

A professor once related to a medical school class the three "Ds" of medicine. "The three D's are Diagnosis, Diagnosis and Diagnosis." During the ascendancy of evidence-based medicine, it has become clear that studies of diagnostic tests—be they laboratory tests, imaging procedures, or activities in the examination room—have been of poor quality. The development of evidence-based guidelines related to diagnostic testing is thus made more difficult by the poor quality of the underlying studies, but the tools of evidence-based medicine can be brought together in this key effort to actually affect patient care.

For guidelines to be useful, they must be developed by a serious, sustained effort of a multidisciplinary team of individuals who understand not only the relevant medical and laboratory issues, but also the principles of evidence-based medicine. Laboratorians must be involved in these teams. Laboratorians are critical in explaining not only the facts of tests that are relevant to the guideline but also the principles of laboratory medicine. Laboratorians must meld those facts and principles with the powerful tools of evidence-based medicine so that guidelines can serve the true goal of evidence-based medicine to improve the care of the individual patient. Despite the challenges, it can be done.

APPENDIX 1

Annotated additional reading

Reading
- Shaneyfelt TM, Mayo-Smith MF, Rothwangl J. Are guidelines following guidelines? The methodological quality of clinical practice guidelines in the peer-reviewed medical literature. J Am Med Assoc 1999;281:1900–5.
  Evidence is not used well in guidelines.
- Haycox A, Bagust A, Walley T. Clinical guidelines—the hidden costs. Br Med J 1999;318:391–3.
  Evidence from the controlled environment of a randomized controlled trial may not be reproducible.

- Harbour R, Miller J. A new system for grading recommendations in evidence based guidelines. Br Med J 2001;323:334–6.
  A thoughtful look at grading that considers the possibility that the best evidence may not be from a randomized controlled trial.
- A guide to the development, implementation and evaluation of clinical practice guidelines. National Health and Medical Research Council (NHMRC) Endorsed 16 November 1998, ISBN 1864960485.
  http://www.health.gov.au/nhmrc/publications/pdf/cp30.pdf (accessed March 29, 2003)
  A detailed and comprehensive guide with an excellent section on techniques for dissemination and implementation of guidelines in Australia.
- *A Guideline Developer's Handbook.* Scottish Intercollegiate Guidelines Network.
  Published February 2001, last updated October 2002 (but dated November 2002).
  http://www.sign.ac.uk/guidelines/fulltext/50/index.html (accessed March 29, 2003)
  An up-to-date document with checklists and tools for continuing professional development for developers of guidelines.
- Eccles M, Mason J. How to develop cost-conscious guidelines. Health Technol Assess 2001;5:1–69. Full text available (without charge) at http://www.ncchta.org/fullmono/mon516.pdf
  As the title implies, this addresses costs more than do the other guidance documents.
- Roe MT, Ohman EM, Pollack CV, Peterson ED, Brandis RG, Harrington RA, et al. Changing the model of care for patients with acute coronary syndromes. Am Heart J (In press).
  Provides useful guidance on implementation of guidelines.

APPENDIX 2

Annotated list of additional web sites

www.agreecollaboration.org
AGREE is an international collaboration of researchers and policy makers who seek to improve the quality and effectiveness of clinical practice guidelines by establishing a shared framework for their development, reporting and assessment.

www.ahcpr.gov/
The health services research arm of the U.S. Department of Health and Human Services (HHS), complementing the biomedical research mission of its sister agency, the National Institutes of Health. Supporting Evidence-based Practice Centers that review and synthesize scientific evidence for conditions or technologies that are costly, common, or important to the Medicare or Medicaid programs.

www.guidelines-international.net
The Guidelines International Network (G-I-N) is a major new international
initiative involving organizations from around the world. G-I-N seeks to improve
the quality of health care by promoting systematic development of clinical
practice guidelines and their application into practice.

www.york.ac.uk/inst/crd/
The Centre for Reviews and Dissemination (CRD) was established in January
1994 to provide the NHS with important information on the effectiveness of
treatments and the delivery and organisation of health care. CRD is intended to
promote research-based practice in the NHS by offering rigorous and systematic
reviews on selected topics, a database of good quality reviews, a dissemination
service and an information service.

www.nice.org.uk/
The National Institute for Clinical Excellence (NICE) was set up as a Special
Health Authority for England and Wales on April 1, 1999. It is part of the
National Health Service (NHS), and its role is to provide patients, health
professionals, and the public with authoritative, robust and reliable guidance on
current "best practice." The guidance will cover both individual health
technologies (including medicines, medical devices, diagnostic techniques, and
procedures) and the clinical management of specific conditions.

www.sign.ac.uk/
The Scottish Intercollegiate Guidelines Network (SIGN) was formed in 1993. Its
objective is to improve the quality of healthcare for patients in Scotland by
reducing variation in practice and outcome, through the development and
dissemination of national clinical guidelines containing recommendations for
effective practice based on current evidence.

REFERENCES

1. Institute of Medicine. Clinical Practice Guidelines: Directions for a New
   Program, Field MJ, Lohr KN, eds. Washington, DC: National Academy Press,
   1990:38.
2. Dufour DR, Lott JA, Nolte FS, Gretch DR, Koff RS, Seeff LB. Diagnosis and
   monitoring of hepatic injury. II. Recommendations for use of laboratory tests
   in screening, diagnosis, and monitoring. Clin Chem 2000;46:2050–68.
3. Sacks DB, Bruns DE, Goldstein DE, Maclaren NK, McDonald JM, Parrott M.
   Guidelines and recommendations for laboratory analysis in the diagnosis and
   management of diabetes mellitus. Clin Chem 2002;48:436–72.
4. Briss PA, Zaza S, Pappaioanou M, Fielding J, Wright-De Aguero L, Truman
   BI, et al. Developing an evidence-based guide to community preventive
   services—methods. The Task Force on Community Preventive Services. Am J
   Prev Med 2000;18(1 Suppl):35–43.
5. Woolf SH, George JN. Evidence-based medicine. Interpreting studies and
   setting policy. Hematol Oncol Clin North Am 2000;14:761–84.

6. Shekelle PG, Woolf SH, Eccles M, Grimshaw J. Clinical guidelines: developing guidelines. Br Med J 1999;318:593–6.
7. Kost GJ. National Guideline Clearinghouse. URL: www.guideline.gov/index. asp. Clin Chem 2000;46:141–2 [Web site review].
8. Leape LL, Park RE, Kahan JP, Brook RH. Group judgments of appropriateness: the effect of panel composition. Qual Assur Health Care 1992;4:151–9.
9. Bossuyt PM, Lijmer JG, Mol BW. Randomised comparisons of medical tests: sometimes invalid, not always efficient. Lancet 2000;356:1844–7.
10. Fraser CG, Petersen PH. Analytical performance characteristics should be judged against objective quality specifications. Clin Chem 1999;45:321–3.
11. Klee GG, Schryver PG, Kisabeth RM. Analytic bias specifications based on the analysis of effects on performance of medical guidelines. Scand J Clin Lab Invest 1999;59:509–12.
12. Boyd JC, Bruns DE. Quality specifications for glucose meters: assessment by simulation modeling of errors in insulin dose. Clin Chem 2001;47:209–14.
13. van Wijk MA, van der Lei J, Mosseveld M, Bohnen AM, van Bemmel JH. Compliance of general practitioners with a guideline-based decision support system for ordering blood tests. Clin Chem 2002;48:55–60.
14. Shekelle PG, Ortiz E, Rhodes S, Morton SC, Eccles MP, Grimshaw JM, et al. Validity of the Agency for Healthcare Research and Quality clinical practice guidelines: how quickly do guidelines become outdated? J Am Med Assoc 2001;286:1461–7.
15. Feder G, Eccles M, Grol R, Griffiths C, Grimshaw J. Clinical guidelines: using clinical guidelines. Br Med J 1999;318:728–30.
16. Implementing clinical practice guidelines. Margolis CZ, Cretin S, eds. Chicago, IL: American Hospital Association Press, 1999:223pp.

11

The Role of Clinical Audit

Julian H. Barth

"Hallo!" said Piglet, "what are you doing?"
"Hunting," said Pooh.
"Hunting what?"
"Tracking something," said Winnie-the-Pooh very mysteriously.
"Tracking what" said Piglet, coming closer.
"That's just what I ask myself. I ask myself, What?"
"What do you think you'll answer?"
"I shall have to wait until I catch up with it" said Winnie-the-Pooh.
　　　　　　　　　—Winnie-the-Pooh. A.A. Milne, 1926

Laboratory medicine was one of the first areas in clinical medicine to embrace the widespread use of audit. This reflective process undoubtedly contributed to the improvement in the standard of laboratory analyses and has been enhanced by the uptake of external as well as internal quality assurance. External quality assurance (EQA) has been continuously refined and is now accepted as a routine component of laboratory practice. Moreover, it is embraced by technologists and managers alike, which ensures that problems are not only rapidly identified but proactively sought and actively rectified. EQA has continued to evolve and over recent years, some schemes, notably UK NEQAS, has introduced exercises to evaluate interpretative and investigative strategies of laboratories.

Clinical audit is the next step in the process of ensuring that laboratories provide accurate useful investigations for clinical care. This phase is being driven both by the evidence-based philosophy of 21st century medicine and also by the near universal need to provide the most cost-effective services. The funding position of laboratory medicine throughout the world is becoming critical. Over the past few decades, this problem has been approached by the use of increasing levels of automation and the use of discretionary test groups rather than indiscriminate profiles. At the same time, attempts have been made to improve clinicians' use of laboratories; but this is quite labor intensive and only provides small benefits (1, 2). The next process in improving laboratory usage will be through electronic requesting linked to intelligent systems. However, these systems will need to be designed with appropriate guidelines and these will need to be continuously evaluated and updated. Other chapters cover the issues of the guideline development that embraces the evidence for laboratory testing. This chapter will cover the issues of determining best practice and quality improvement through clinical audit.

CLINICAL AUDIT

Clinical audit is a process of measuring clinical procedures and outcomes in order to improve practice. Audit might best be defined by comparison with clinical research: research is concerned with discovering the "right thing to do," whereas audit is concerned with ensuring that it is "done right." The involvement of audit in the quality improvement cycle (Figure 1) comes after the development of standards of clinical practice (investigation or treatment) and is used for the assessment of how well the guidelines are followed in order to validate clinical care.

There are two main forms of audit; the first is aimed at solving problems in either process or outcome. Typical examples might be the exploration of factors that delay turnaround times or inconsistency in sample timing of dynamic endocrine tests. This type of audit requires the identification of rate-limiting steps and needs imagination and inquisitiveness rather than precise scientific evaluation. The second form of audit involves a more systematic approach to a clinical area. In the first stage, it may be determining practice or adherence to guidelines (if these exist). In either case, a very clear objective needs to be formulated in advance and data need to be collected in a formal and exact manner to answer the question. Both forms of clinical audit should be subject to formal evaluation to determine the effectiveness and cost of the practice. This latter step is important because it is critical that audit becomes part of institutional organization in order to ensure that its findings are incorporated into everyday practice.

Good clinical audit is probably also a powerful tool for physician education/behavior modification. The results from evidence-based reviews are not supportive of this concept (2) but this may be due to the paucity of studies. Certainly the simplistic approach of laboratories trying to educate by sending out notifications of over- or underutilization of tests to physicians has little impact. However, the data starting to emerge from systematic audits of clinical practice in cardiac care are encouraging (3, 4).

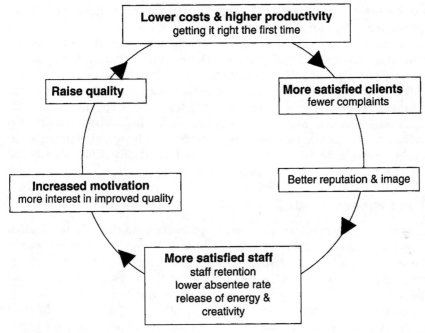

Figure 1 Quality improvement cycle.

Why?

There are clearly political and professional reasons for the implementation of clinical audit. First, there is political concern at the variation in standards and outcomes of clinical practice across the country. It is hoped that audit will explore the reasons for some areas having above average outcomes and what factors lead to poor outcomes in other areas. It should not, however, be immediately anticipated that any improvements will be associated with cost savings. Audit may well reveal shortcomings initially introduced as cost measures. Second, one major benefit of clinical audit is the potential for improving professional job satisfaction.

The commitment to audit and, therefore, quality assurance (QA) will help uphold professional standards and ultimately result in fewer dissatisfied patients and clinical colleagues. On an individual level, it should lead to:

- increased job satisfaction,
- an opportunity for continual improvement,
- recognition of achievements.
- productive use of time and effort by removal of inefficient practice, and
- the acquisition of new skills and experience.

These are, of course, all the components and benefits of appropriate continuing professional development.

A further value of clinical audit is to build onto the evidence created by randomized controlled trials (RCTs). These trials are performed by an extremely rigid methodology that demands narrow patient-entry requirements. This results in a case mix that is likely to be quite unrepresentative of normal clinical experience. However, the trials are used to establish primary guidelines. The *importance of clinical audit with outcome evaluation* is to determine whether the guidelines generated by these, often pharmaceutically driven, trials are valid for normal clinical practice. Clinical audit can then fill the gap between research and reality (5).

The Process of Audit

Several related activities are encompassed by the term clinical audit, including routine data collection, surveys, and complete audit cycles. However, these processes by themselves do not constitute real audit because there is no commitment to act on the findings and institute change. Some surveys will identify variations in practice that cannot be moved forward because no standards can be agreed upon, e.g., urea and electrolyte profiles (6). This should not be taken to denigrate the acquisition of data since this action alone does initiate inquisitiveness and therefore has the potential to induce change in practice as can been seen in the following situation.

Example 1: In the Newcastle region of Northern England, there were 15 laboratories with four different methods for the measurement of glycated hemoglobin (HbA1c). Since there is currently no standard for HbA1c, these laboratories were providing different HbA1c values, which created difficulties for clinicians who desired to use the clinical targets established by the Diabetes Control and Complications Trial (DCCT). This was particularly problematic for clinicians who served several hospitals with different methods. In order to try to standardize the measurement of HbA1c, Gibb et al. (7) distributed samples to all laboratories. All samples were simultaneously calibrated by the central biochemistry laboratory of the DCCT research group at the University of Minnesota.

The samples were from 50 diabetic and nondiabetic subjects. They were distributed in two batches with a 2-week interval. The mean coefficient of variation (CV) for these results was 15.3% (95% CI 14.0–16.5). Using a regression equation relating a subset of seven of these results to their assigned reference values, the authors calculated a glycated hemoglobin index for all of the other samples distributed. Following distribution, the mean interlaboratory CV improved to 4.6% (95% CI 4.0–5.1), p<0.0001. The percentage bias of results from the reference method also improved from 15.1% (95% CI 9.4–20.1) to 4.67% (95% CI 4.05–5.25) after alignment, p<0.001. The authors demon-

*strated that considerable method- related differences can be reduced by em-
ploying a simple strategy of distributing appropriately calibrated samples.
Moreover, considerable clinical benefit can be obtained if the methods are
calibrated to those methods with extensive clinical interpretative evidence,
such as in this experiment with DCCT.*

The complete audit cycle consists of a number of processes, which include setting standards, observing, evaluating, reporting, and making
changes prior to starting again (Figure 2). The All Wales Audit Group gives
an excellent demonstration of the use of clinical audit in laboratory medicine (8).

Choosing a Topic

The performance of good audit is as challenging as good research and pos-
ing appropriate questions is equally important. The process of selecting important questions will include whether it is worthwhile, measurable, and
achievable. If these parameters cannot be realized or the question cannot
be clearly defined, the topic should be abandoned and another area should
be explored. Audit projects are expensive and can only be justified if there
is a measurable benefit to patient care. The following example illustrates a
case where an initial survey was performed for a complex problem, that of
excessive inappropriate in-patient laboratory investigations.

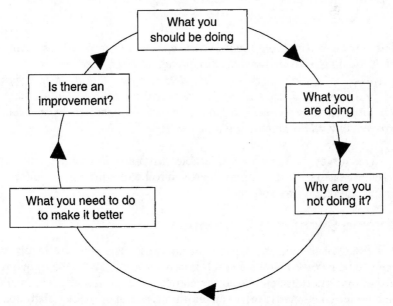

Figure 2 The audit cycle described with practical everyday terms!

Example 2: *The authors studied the pattern of clinical requests for thyroid function tests (TFTs) in hospital inpatients by combining data from the laboratory and clinical information systems. All information on TFTs requested from April to August 1996 was collected; collected information included patient demographics, location, and requesting consultant. This information was then merged with data regarding individual consultant workload and the diagnostic (ICD-10) codes for each inpatient.*

TFTs were defined as abnormal if either the TSH was greater than 6 IU/L or both the total T4 was greater than 12.4 µg/dL (>160 nmol/L) and TSH was less than 0.05 IU/L; these values were chosen to exclude patients on appropriate thyroxine replacement therapy (in-house data). Repeat samples were defined as those tests repeated on any patient under a single consultant within 14 days of a previous test.

The total number of TFTs performed on 30,393 in-patient episodes during the study period was 1725. Diagnostic codes related to thyroid and/or pituitary disease were present in 273 episodes. Data were excluded on 302 patients in whom no information on the requesting consultant was available. Of these latter tests, 54% were performed in the acute medical admission ward.

The overall rate of testing thyroid function was 5.7%. Abnormalities in thyroid function tests were found in 1% of the inpatients tested. The median rate of abnormalities in TFTs per consultant-team was 0.48% (range 0–12%; 25–75 centile values 0–1.4). There was, however, considerable variation in testing rates (Figure 3).

This approach to auditing clinical practice shows the power of combining different databases from separate disciplines. It confirmed the considerable prevalence of testing for thyroid disorders and also that the teams with the lowest disease incidence had the lowest diagnostic hit-rate. Unfortunately, it was not possible to reconcile difference in attitudes between clinicians and no progress toward a standard could be developed.

The survey confirmed considerable variability in practice but the underlying reasons for this variation proved to be too difficult to address and no further action was possible.

Gaining Support of Colleagues

It is essential to gain the support of all individuals who are involved, or likely to be involved, in the audit. It is easy to be glib about the frequent use of the term multidisciplinary in the context of clinical audit. The reality is that modern medicine involves an enormous raft of professional groups and

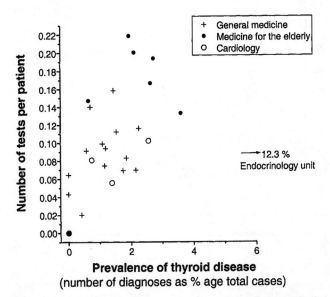

Figure 3 Example 2—Comparison of incidence of TFT testing (total number of tests/total number of subjects) with disease prevalence in hospital in patients.

unless they are all involved in the audit, then its conclusions will not necessarily be implemented. As illustrated in Example 3, audits that are performed without including the clinical unit into ownership of the project frequently result in little apparent benefit.

Example 3: In 1999, following a leading article in the British Medical Journal on hyponatremia in orthopedic wards, the authors performed a search of the biochemistry laboratory computer for sodium measurements on patients in the orthopedic wards. Data on sodium values collected over a 5-month period were collected. This information was prepared as a graph demonstrating the frequency distribution of sodium values and was given to the lead clinician for orthopedics. The apparent result was that a clinical protocol was drawn up to manage these patients. No further involvement was made by the laboratory. Three years later, in a pique of curiosity, the issue of orthopedic hyponatremia was again explored by the laboratory. A further search of an equivalent 5-month period was made. The pattern of hyponatremia for both periods is illustrated in Figure 4. It can be seen that, apart from an increase in workload from the orthopedic unit, the pattern of hyponatremia is essentially unchanged. This outcome should have been quite predictable since the audit was performed without the active participation of all parties and no elements of the clinical management team were involved in the process except as recipients of unrequested data.

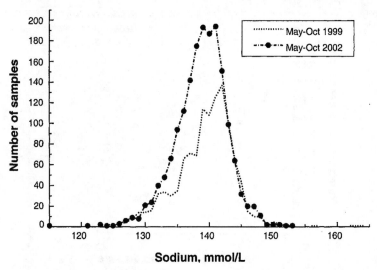

Figure 4 Example 3—Distribution of plasma sodium measurements in orthopedic wards in two 6-month periods.

Develop Standards

Once the question has been posed, it is necessary to establish correct practice. This is traditionally performed by literature searches (*see* chapters 6 and 8–10). Important questions are likely to have been considered by others who may have already prepared guidelines that can be used. These are not always easily found as they may have been prepared by another professional group without any laboratory medicine involvement. The searches should include professional societies web sites.

There may not be any evidence to answer your question. In this case, either convene a group of experts to provide a consensus on best practice, or alternatively it may be appropriate to perform a survey of current practice (*see* Figure 1). This survey can help to define a baseline from which standards can be established and subsequently audited as seen in the following example of a successful audit.

Example 4: *An extensive survey of laboratory endocrine practice was performed in 1995 (9). This illustrated how widely divergent practices were throughout the United Kingdom. In response to these findings, the Association of Clinical Biochemists (ACB) convened a meeting of all interested laboratory endocrinologists to consider how best to proceed. One of the outcomes was the commissioning of (in those days) a non-systematic review of the low dose (overnight) dexamethasone suppression test for the diagnosis of Cushing's disease. This was necessary as many respondents of the original survey did not have a clear idea of how much serum cortisol should be suppressed during this diagnostic test. The survey and the subsequent review (10) were published in the Annals of Clinical Biochemistry in 1995 and 1997, respectively. The review concluded that the low dose (overnight) dexamethasone suppression test could be used as a screening test for Cushing's disease. The recommended protocol was 1 mg taken at 11 p.m. and plasma/serum cortisol taken at 9 a.m. the following day. The recommended dose of dexamethasone was 1 mg and the cutoff for a positive test for cortisol was 1.8 µg/dL (50 nmol/L).*

A follow-up survey was recirculated throughout clinical laboratories in the United Kingdom in 2003. The same questions regarding the low-dose (overnight) dexamethasone suppression test were used. The population approached was probably similar, although different mailing lists were used; in 1995, heads of departments were included using the ACB mailing list, whereas in 2002, quality officers were included using the United Kingdom National External Quality Assurance Scheme lists. The responses for the dexamethasone suppression test were similar with 48 and 51% returns, respectively, in the two surveys.

The results of both surveys' question on the cut-off value for 9 a.m. cortisol are shown in Figure 5. It can be seen that in the first survey 20.4% reported a

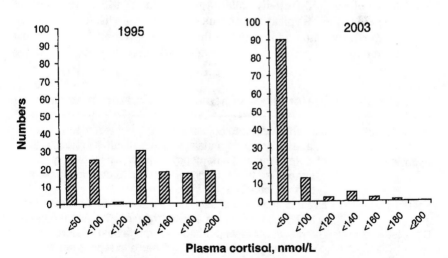

Figure 5 Example 4—Distribution of responses to audit questionnaires on the 9 a.m. cortisol value that would exclude Cushing's disease after an overnight dexamethasone suppression test. The second questionnaire was distributed after publication of a guideline.

cut-off value less than 1.8 μg/dL (<50nmol/L) whereas in 2002, this had increased to 79.6%. Moreover, a dose of 1 mg was recommended by 69% in 1995 and 89% in the later survey.

An important component of a standard is the means and strategy of measurement of that standard and a definition of this measurement must be made first, whether the standard is a process or clinical outcome.

Project Management

The multidisciplinary group involved in the audit will need to decide who is performing the audit. This aspect is clearly obvious for national or regional projects, indeed, a team may be required for these. However, even for local audits, appropriate individuals must be chosen in order to ensure that this exercise is not threatening to any member of the group.

Methods

Audit measures current practice. The methods used do not change practice and any intervention that does change practice should be the consequence of the audit process. Therefore, audit methods do not typically involve randomization, use of control groups, or placebo (*see* Audit or Research section). The main methods used in clinical audit are direct observation, checklists, documentation audit, questionnaires, interviews, and case reviews. The choice of method (usually called a tool in audit) will depend on the question being asked. Typical performance indicators are listed in Table 1.

It is worth spending time ensuring that the chosen methods are robust and that measurable parameters are selected whether they are qualitative

Table 1
Types of clinical performance indicators in laboratory medicine[a]

Preanalytical	Demand (workload/population), range of test menu, laboratory user manuals, and investigative protocols
Analytical	Mix of routine and emergency tests, within laboratory turnaround times, quality assurance at decision-making concentrations
Postanalytical	Evaluation of clinical decisions made on basis of laboratory tests, laboratory data availability, mortality, and morbidity
Complete process	Range/cost of tests per bed-day, range/cost of tests per diagnostic group/diagnosis, "needle to report" turnaround times, user satisfaction, resource used

[a]Performance indicators are arranged in a classical laboratory style but could alternatively be based on a different structure, e.g., activity, costs, structure, process, outputs, or outcome.

or quantitative. The next step is method evaluation. This is standard practice in research projects and should equally be part of audit projects. A questionnaire can be piloted with a few colleagues. Data collection fields can be evaluated with a few cases. It is much easier to correct a poorly designed questionnaire or data collection form than to try to interpret muddled or incomplete data sets at the end of the data collection phase.

Collecting, Monitoring, and Reviewing Data

The aim of performing an audit is to improve clinical care. Therefore, during the process of data collection, the data should be examined to determine whether there are obvious aspects of the process that are faulty. These can be rectified immediately. One blunder is enough—there is no need to collect sufficient to reach statistical significance. However, the situation when monitoring guidelines is different and begs the question "What makes a guideline invalid?" A single case that highlights an important exception that has not been mentioned may merit a change, e.g., an important drug contraindication that has not been mentioned in the guideline. In contrast, a large number of poor outcomes may not mean that the guideline should be changed. In the situation where a guideline recommends offering amniocentesis for pregnant women identified as having a high risk of having a child with Down's syndrome, there are likely to be miscarriages caused by the procedure. However, these outcomes do not necessarily make the guideline wrong. Of course, the guideline should suggest that women receive information on the potential risk, and the risk should have been taken into account when formulating the guideline, but the poor outcomes do not necessarily invalidate the guideline.

There are a number of large-scale clinical audit databases providing an overview of regional or national clinical practice. These databases provide evidence of ongoing data collection, monitoring, data review, and feedback of results to users for process improvement. Examples in the United Kingdom include the Renal Register (11), Myocardial Infarction National Audit Project (MINAP) (12), and Quality Indicators for Diabetes Services (QUIDS). Examples in the United States include the American Heart Association "Get with the guidelines" program (3) and CRUSADE (Can Rapid Risk Stratification of Unstable Angina Patients Suppress ADverse Outcomes with Early Implementation of the ACC/AHA Guidelines) (4). Other large-scale audits closer to the laboratory include annual reports by EQA schemes but these are not openly available to nonparticipants.

Analysis and Implementation

On completion of the collection process, the data can be fully analyzed to answer the original question. A well-designed audit will identify the stages in the process that are functioning poorly and well and some that may be rate limiting. All these areas need to be identified so that the good parts can be complimented and the poorly functioning and rate-limiting steps can be improved. These will require a formal action plan to ensure that resources can be directed to make the necessary improvements. These improvements will themselves need to be audited, first, to ensure that they are implemented and second, to ensure that implementation was the appropriate step. Example 5 illustrates a successful small management change (request card design) that has had profound effects but it can be seen that there are the beginnings of a relapse in the effects and a new intervention is required.

Example 5: Normal clinical practice allows physicians complete freedom to choose laboratory investigations. The authors noted considerable variation in requesting endocrine tests by physicians in the gynecology endocrine clinic. Investigative guidelines were developed with the gynecology specialists for the most appropriate tests (13). These were cascaded to the clinical staff in seminars and by posting the recommendations in the out-patient clinic. A request card was specially designed with "tick-boxes" based on clinical conditions (e.g., hirsutism, PCO, infertility), but no specific tests were named. These were designed to help clinical staff adhere to the agreed investigative protocols. Each clinician was given the freedom to tick a box or to choose other patterns of tests.

The workload was assessed for a 2-year period before and after the introduction of these cards. The clinical caseload remained steady with an unchanged case mix at a median of 227 cases per month. The numbers of all endocrine tests, except progesterone and SHBG, fell by 19% ($p<0.0001$).

This long-term monitoring of workload demonstrates the variability in monthly testing but that appropriately introduced guidelines show an immediate effect (Figure 6). However, regular monitoring and feedback are required to maintain the impetus of the original aim which, in this case, was to make the tests fit the case.

Infrastructure for Clinical Audit

Clinical audit can be performed in isolation. However, this approach will limit its ability to provide significant widescale changes because of the multiplicity of processes involved in clinical care. In view of this complexity, audit is most valuable when it is applied by someone with an overview of the whole process of clinical care. This allows it to be used in the most efficient way to solve problem areas and ease bottlenecks. In order for this to occur, audit needs to be embedded as part of the management process. This integration means that ownership of the findings belongs to the organization and the solutions are more likely to be implemented. Analytical quality as-

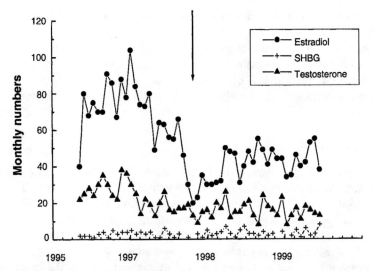

Figure 6 Example 5—Workload distribution for some endocrine tests in a gynecology-endocrine clinic before and after the introduction (arrow) of a disease-based request card.

surance is a perfect model to show the benefit of this integration. It also shows that correctly applied audit will be supported and encouraged by management who will see that the resources for audit are well used.

A further component of successful audit is its use within a nonthreatening and equitable environment. No one is willing to expose their professional practice in an environment that espouses a blame culture!

Clinical audit is usually expected to include some patient input. It is unclear at present whether methods in laboratory-based clinical audit are sufficiently well developed for patient input to be useful. It is clear that there should be links to postgraduate education units to ensure that the audit information is disseminated to clinical staff by the best available means.

Guidelines for Success

Successful audit is a result of commitment by involved staff. Colleagues and other staff are best kept involved if they are included in the design and implementation of the audit and feel that their professional judgment has been included. Other important factors include the relevance of the project to the local environment and, while specific data may remain confidential, the overall results should be freely communicated to all participants. Larger scale projects need the same factors to retain commitment but will involve larger teams making project planning and management as well as the dissemination of results more important. Regional and national projects require teams of audit officers who will need to be adequately trained, supported, and resourced.

A sign of the successful incorporation of clinical audit is the development of a culture of questioning, continuing evaluation, and improvement of clinical effectiveness. While this should be focused on patient outcomes, it is likely that laboratory medicine will continue to use surrogate markers (14).

Barriers to Success

It is important to recognize the factors that will impede progress. Most of these are the converse of the factors indicated to predict success. The most important is poor communication between members of the team. These include the principal leaders, collaborating clinicians, managers, and data handlers. A failure of communication will result in poor progress due to a lack of awareness of the guidelines, disagreement with them, or merely uncertainty of their value. Overall, it will mean that established practice will not be modified. Lack of feedback will also act as a barrier to change. Poor communication is a failure on behalf of the project leadership. Other factors will include lack of expertise in project design and analysis, and external factors such as time constraints, lack of resources, and lack of reminders.

AUDIT OR RESEARCH AND ETHICS

Research projects require ethical approval, and there is a narrow dividing line between audit and research. In general, audit can be described as a process that does not cause any disturbance to patients beyond that required for clinical management. Audit should not cause any risk to patients. Risk in this context should be used in its broadest sense and should include significant invasion of privacy or the imposition of a burden beyond that experienced in routine care. Audit does not typically involve randomization, use of control groups, or placebo. Good audit projects require the same preparatory work as good research projects and, if in any doubt, one would be well advised to seek advice from a clinical ethics research committee prior to starting an audit project.

In the United States, Heath Insurance Portability and Accountability Act (HIPAA) regulations have added a new dimension to ethics, privacy, and access to patient information. Information used for research purposes must have either a waiver from the Institutional Review Board and/or written patient authorization prior to examination of records and data. However, access to protected health information for the purposes of treatment, payment, or operations is not covered by the stringent HIPAA regulations. The clinical audit function should be considered a part of "operations" in most cases.

SUMMARY

Clinical audit is a process used to assess how well patient care is performed. The benefits of a well-performed audit are felt by the patient and also by the professional teams. Staff involved in the care of patients benefit when they can see or be shown that their individual contributions are being effective. Audit works best when all participants are involved in the planning and design of the projects. However, the most important contribution is by the involvement of management as only they can ensure that identified problems can and will be rectified. Optimal laboratory practice will occur when clinical audit is as securely embedded into laboratory procedure as analytical quality assurance.

REFERENCES[a]

1. Fraser CG, Woodford FP. Strategies to modify the test-requesting patterns of clinicians. Ann Clin Biochem 1987;24:223–31.
2. Thomson O'Brien MA, Oxman AD, David DA, Haynes RB, Freemantle N, Harvey EL. Audit and feedback: effects on professional practice and health care outcomes (Cochrane review). In: The Cochrane Library, issue 4, 2002. Oxford: Update Software.
3. American Heart Association "Get with the guidelines" program http://www.americanheart.org/presenter.jhtml?identifier=699 (accessed April 2, 2003).
4. CRUSADE http://www.crusadeqi.com/ (accessed April 2, 2003).
5. Bero LA, Grilli R, Grimshaw JM, Harvey E, Oxman AD, Thomson MA. Closing the gap between research and practice: an overview of systematic reviews of interventions to promote the implementation of research findings. Br Med J 1998;317:465–8.
6. Broughton PMG, Worthington DJ. Laboratories respond differently to the same clinical request. Ann Clin Biochem 1989;26:119–21.
7. Gibb I, Parnham AJ, Lord C, Steffes MW, Bucksa J, Marshall S. Standardization of glycated haemoglobin assays throughout the Northern region of England: a pilot study. Diab Med 1997;14:584–8.
8. Wales Audit Group (http://www.acb.org.uk/welshaudit) (accessed April 6, 2003).
9. Barth JH, Seth J, Howlett TA, Freedman DB. A survey of endocrine function testing by clinical biochemistry laboratories in the UK. Ann Clin Biochem 1995;32:442–9.
10. Wood PJ, Barth JH, Freedman DB, Perry L, Sheridan B. Evidence for the low dose dexamethasone suppression test to screen for Cushing's syndrome—recommendations for a protocol for UK biochemistry laboratories. Ann Clin Biochem 1997;34:222–9.

[a]For additional information, readers might wish to consult: Best Practice in Clinical Audit http://www.nelh.nhs.uk/nice_bpca/pbca.htm (accessed March 30, 2003) and Pruce D, Aggarwal R. *National clinical audits: a handbook for good practice*. London: Royal College of Physicians, 2000.

11. The UK Renal Registry (http://www.renalreg.com/home.htm) (accessed April 2, 2003).
12. MINAP (http://www.rcplondon.ac.uk/college/ceeu/ceeu_ami_home.htm) (accessed April 2, 2003).
13. Barth JH, Balen AH, Jennings A. Appropriate design of biochemistry request cards can promote the use of protocols and reduce unnecessary investigations. Ann Clin Biochem 2001;38:714–6.
14. Waise A, Plebani M. Which surrogate marker can be used to assess the effectiveness of the laboratory and its contribution to clinical outcome? Ann Clin Biochem 2001;38:589–95.

12

Teaching Evidence-Based Laboratory Medicine: A Cultural Experience

Christopher P. Price and Robert H. Christenson

The definition of evidence-based-medicine (EBM) and evidence-based practice proposed by Sackett et al. (1) is generally acknowledged to be definitive and offers great clarity of purpose. This definition describes "the conscientious, explicit and judicious use of best evidence for making decisions about the care of patients," and describes the integration of best research evidence with clinical expertise and patient values. As has been pointed out in earlier chapters, these definitions encompass all of the attitudes, skills, and experience needed to establish and maintain an EBM culture focused on the highest possible quality of care to the patient. By implication, the principles of evidence-based practice are applicable across the breadth of healthcare, throughout the life of the patient, and span the career of the healthcare professional. Thus, the practice of EBM can also be described as problem-based, lifelong learning (2).

Instilling the culture of EBM should begin at the outset of training for the healthcare professional. Indeed as the philosophy of patient empowerment gains momentum, this culture can be introduced into health education initiatives and personal healthcare. Sadly, it is well known that professional performance deteriorates with age and, together with advances in knowledge and technology, this renders continuing education an essential feature of ensuring that the ideal is maintained (3, 4).

Teaching EBM is therefore applicable to the trainee healthcare professional, as well as to the registered practitioner, initially in developing the right skills to establish good practice; in gaining experience; and then maintaining expertise, gaining new skills, and keeping up to date with developments in the field. One element of the definition given earlier refers to "best evidence" and the teaching of EBM principles applies equally to:

- the researcher developing new evidence,
- the evaluator reviewing the evidence,
- the teacher or facilitator disseminating the evidence, and
- the practitioner using the evidence.

Importantly the culture of evidence-based practice is equally applicable to the spectrum of healthcare professionals at all levels of involvement or contact with the patient. It is worth emphasizing again that EBM practice focuses on the individual patient. Thus, there will be a core curriculum and set of learning tools that will be supplemented to accommodate different learning settings and varying objectives in the areas of research, dissemination of information, and routine practice.

This philosophy is undoubtedly applicable to laboratory medicine, although—perhaps a little unusually—some observers question the existence of a tangible link between the laboratorian and the patient. Note the term tangible, because there is no doubt a paradox here in that many clinicians, nurses, and patients see the laboratory as a means of generating numbers and opinions, while others believe that involvement of laboratorians in their day-to-day clinical decision making is essential. Whose responsibility is it to ensure that the number and/or opinion is correctly and/or effectively utilized in the care of the patient? In the United Kingdom with the advent of Clinical Governance, it could be argued that this would ultimately be the responsibility of the Chief Executive of the Hospital or Primary Care Trust. In exercising this responsibility, the Chief Executive will want to be assured that the clinician and the laboratorian are working together in the best interest of the patient and would expect to be informed if there was not clinical compliance with laboratory guidelines. Data on the incorrect or ineffective use of laboratory data are often anecdotal and definitive examples are rarely published in the peer-reviewed literature, although they are often catalogued in the reports of medical litigation cases. There are, however, some examples (5–7) that can point to where effort is required to improve the effectiveness of tests. The routine commitment to regular clinical audit, an integral part of Clinical Governance and quality assurance, will also identify where compliance with best practice is lacking and where there is opportunity for improvement (chapter 11).

A review of the laboratory medicine services in the United Kingdom in the mid-1990s pointed to the role of the laboratory staff in the education and training of the users of the service as well as in clinical audit (8). However, there is little evidence from audit and benchmarking activities and the definition of performance indicators that the effectiveness of the laboratory service is assessed in terms of patient outcomes.

This chapter applies the thinking on EBM teaching to laboratory medicine. The laboratory is clearly one member of the team responsible for care of the patient, and therefore the approach emphasizes the importance of integration and harmonization. Harmonization is essential for ensuring communication, and use of a "common language," as well as for sharing resources. Integration is important because the laboratory is part of the team and should operate in the spirit of actively identifying and providing services to meet the needs of the patient and the clinician. The product of the laboratory should therefore be seen as part of a seamless continuum of information with the interpretation of results taking into account other relevant preanalytical and technical factors. It is an interesting aside to ponder on whether point-of-care testing (POCT) achieves this integration more successfully, bringing a unique value to this approach.

This chapter relies heavily on the writing of Sackett et al. (9) and will apply the thinking of these pioneers to the realm of the laboratorian.

GENERAL PHILOSOPHY

Sackett et al. (9) identified seven "notions" that they considered important for EBM teaching. These are set out in Table 1 with annotations and additions that are appropriate for the laboratorian.

Patient Centered

Evidence of the clinical utility of a diagnostic test, by its nature, is established on a large population of patients. In laboratory medicine, especially

Table 1
General philosophies on teaching and learning evidence-based (laboratory) medicine

Clinical Medicine	Laboratory Medicine
Teaching and learning evidence-based (laboratory) medicine should:	
• be patient centered	• be patient centered
	• be user centered; appreciate the clinical context and clinical needs
• be learner centered	• be learner centered
• be active and interactive	• be active, proactive, and interactive
• be modeled as essential to becoming an expert clinician	• emphasize the contribution of the clinical team
• take advantage of clinical setting and circumstances	• emphasize the role of the laboratory in making clinical decisions
• be well prepared	• be well prepared
• be multistaged	• be multistaged

where there are high levels of automation and large workloads, it is easy to lose focus on the needs of the individual patient. However, one of the most important issues when using best evidence in the care of patients is to ensure that the evidence is applicable to the unique setting of the individual patient.

Invariably the context of the individual patient helps the practitioner define the clinical question and appraise the applicability of the available evidence. The unique setting must account for the potential impact of confounding factors at the interface between the analytical result and the patient's unique clinical status. These are often referred to as "preanalytical factors" and they are discussed in the context of defining the clinical question in chapter 2.

Clinical decision making must balance the best available evidence with a consideration of risks and benefits, together with an understanding of the patient's preferences (10). The adoption of a patient-centered (or focused) health service requires that, in the case of laboratory medicine, the clinician understands the meaning of the test result, as he/she will be responsible for explaining it to the patient. With the advent of the Internet, it could be argued that this extends to the laboratorian as tools such as LabTestsOnline are accessible to patients (11). Patients are beginning to take more responsibility for their own care and well-being. This change may apply at the level of disease management, e.g., the use of blood glucose testing in the management of diabetes. It may also apply to the choice of intervention to be made after receipt of a set of results, as in the case of the choice of amniocentesis after calculation of the risk score for the detection of Down's syndrome using biochemical markers, or to move to biopsy after receipt of an elevated total prostate-specific antigen result in the case of an asymptomatic man.

Learner Centered

Sackett et al. (9) observed that the learner will vary in terms of initial knowledge base, skill level, learning aptitude, and the effect of competing demands; to appreciate this point, one only has to compare the situation of the newly qualified resident and the specialist with 20 years of practice. This is further emphasized in many ways by considering the learning needs from the perspective of members of the clinical team, which will encompass professionals from very different backgrounds.

The laboratorian will typically gain clinical knowledge and skills from lectures, tutorials, and text resources supplemented with a somewhat passive attendance at some ward rounds or grand rounds. The laboratory knowledge and skills will also be gained from lectures, tutorials, and text resources but this knowledge base will be supplemented with a significant amount of benchwork. In the case of the physician entering laboratory medicine, there will already be some clinical experience using laboratory services and, therefore, presumably experience with critical appraisal of test utilization. Even then it can be argued that this experience will diminish as the laboratory-based physician's focus moves away from the purely clinical environment. In this context, it is interesting to note the trend among clinical pathologists to include an element of direct patient care within their commitments.

This discussion points to the challenge of training each individual team member to ensure the complementarity of knowledge and skill base, to ensure the highest level of team work, and to focus on the patient. This point can be extended to the relationship between the laboratorian and the diagnostic system manufacturer. The analytical characteristics of most assays used in routine practice today are the responsibility of the manufacturer; for this reason, the clinician and the patient are dependent on the relationship between the laboratorian and the supplier. This is sometimes where quality control and assurance schemes break down—in the quality of the dialogue. The parameters of the dialogue are identical in both situations: accurate definition of the problem, critical appraisal of the evidence, and then good communication of the outcome. All too often the evidence is anecdotal without any documentation or data to support a concern and to define exactly the problem at hand. The development and maintenance of new tests and systems depend on continuous, open, and informed dialogue between the manufacturer and the user.

Clinical Context

Chapter 2 covered the importance of a clear understanding of the clinical question; an accurate definition helps to identify the clinical context. Laboratorians are always challenged by the overuse or abuse of testing, the inappropriate testing, and the issue of the appropriate test. An appropriate test has been defined as the test (result) that provides an answer to a clinical question and enables a decision to be made (12, 13). It is then expected that this decision will lead to an action being taken that will deliver an improved health outcome (clinical and/or economic). The latter defines the value of the test.

One of the important aspects of practicing evidence-based (laboratory) medicine is asking answerable questions. As already suggested, if either the question cannot be answered or a decision cannot be made based on receipt of the result, then the test request may be considered inappropriate. Elucidation of the question can sometimes be quite difficult, as has been illustrated in this book. One of the tools used in teaching EBM, which can be applied to laboratory medicine in various different ways, is the "educational prescription" (14).

An outline of the educational prescription as originally described by Sackett et al. (14) is given in Figure 1 adapted for use in laboratory medi-

Patient's Name	Learner (requester)

Clinical question

Context
- Target disorder
- Expected intervention
- Expected outcome

Date and place to be completed

Notes
i.   search strategy
ii. search results
iii. validity of the evidence
iv. importance of this valid evidence
v.   can this evidence be applied to this patient
vi. your evaluation of this process

Figure 1 The educational prescription in laboratory medicine.

cine. It is important to retain the overall structure in order to understand the clinical context and thus the version for laboratory medicine focuses on the diagnostic process, while also attempting to maintain a link to both the clinician and the patient in order to ensure relevance to the final outcome.

This approach to reasoning can be used as an "aide memoire" in a number of situations. The structure of the educational prescription provides the context for the investigation being requested and as the format for the ideal data set when making a request to the laboratory. In order to provide the most effective service, it has often been suggested that the clinical question should be set out first and sent to the laboratory with the specimen, instead of simply ordering a battery of tests. This protocol would allow the laboratorian to analyze the clinical situation, communicate with the caregiver as necessary, and perform the most appropriate tests. This happens already in certain clinical situations where test algorithms and care paths have been established; however, this does not happen in all healthcare systems, especially where test reimbursement is a major determining factor and government regulations prohibit what could be construed as self referral of testing. The most common example where a cascade of tests is performed based on a clinical suspicion or based on an abnormal (sometimes chance) finding is in the case where myeloma is suspected. An elevated total protein may trigger the performance of protein electrophoresis and then immunofixation and monoclonal protein quantitation if an abnormal band is found. There have been other algorithms developed when specific abnormalities are found.

The structure of the educational prescription ensures that the clinical problem is specified, and that the specific question(s) is (are) identified. It recognizes who is responsible for completing the information and at what time, as well as reminding those involved of how to search for and appraise the evidence, together with establishing the relationship with the individual patients' situation. The central element of this process remains establishing the clinical question (15). In the use of any one test, there are likely to be a large number of individual questions, and this provides one of the greatest challenges for the laboratorian in attempting to generate the evidence. The evidence may need to be generated to meet the needs of a number of clinical settings, e.g., patient age, time of day, level of exercise, renal function, and hepatic function, all of which require supplementary interpretation. This might make the response to the educational prescription a rather daunting task, but this is what constitutes "experience."

An important feature of dealing with the wealth of knowledge (evidence) is gathering and maintaining a portfolio of critically appraised topics (CATs). CATs will be discussed later and are described in more detail in chapter 8. They provide a valuable resource for learners and can be readily accessed with modern information technology. Richardson and Burdette (16) recently described the use of a hand-held device for rapidly accessing knowledge databases during a patient consultation; most of the interactions with this system required between 4 and 5 seconds and did not appear to inhibit or delay the consultation process.

Active and Interactive

The essence of being a team player is appreciating and responding to the needs of other team members. This role demands that the laboratorian be "customer focused" and committed to continuing interactive dialogue with clinical colleagues. The question may arise as to who is the customer: does the customer include the patient? In the context of the awareness required, the definition should encompass the patient, the attending clinician, other members of the clinical team, the health service provider, and the policymaker.

Some examples of the importance of adopting an interactive approach are:

- understanding of how, and why, clinicians ask questions
- understanding of the relation between clinical question and test result
- awareness of action prompted by test result
- awareness of relation between test result and outcome
- identification of benefit accruing to patient, clinician and organization
- awareness of quality of evidence

- understanding the specific clinical context
- awareness of confounding factors that might compromise utility
- agreement with local clinical protocol
- compliance with protocol

An interactive and proactive approach is key to successful practice because of the volume of information available to the health professional.

Becoming an Expert Clinician

Sackett et al. (9) stressed that using evidence should be integrated as a fundamental theme or foundation of routine practice, rather than considering it a separate research or governance issue. Thus, the illustration referred to earlier (16) is an important cultural phenomenon to consider. Formulating the question and then the searching for evidence provides a valuable means of building knowledge, confidence, and experience which leads to an enhancement of expertise.

The foundation of evidence is then supplemented by the experience gained from clinical audit (chapter 11), which may lead to a modification of practice as well as providing validation for what might become a clinical protocol, care path, or guideline (chapter 10). It is also important to continue to build on the evidence base; the peer-reviewed literature continues to supply data that can enhance knowledge on the potential utility of diagnostic tests. Assessing the importance of a new test can be a particularly challenging exercise during the early phase of the introduction. However, techniques that continue to build the evidence base will serve to strengthen the confidence in, and define the appropriate use of, the test. In addition, this continuous updating of the database, ideally in real time, will enhance the speed with which experience of the use of the test can be gained. This updating has considerable patient impact, because patients will benefit sooner from the acceptance of the new technology.

Keeping abreast of the literature is something that is second nature to the dedicated researcher; however, the busy practicing healthcare professional cannot always devote the necessary time to this activity. In addition, keeping guidelines up to date is very challenging. It has been suggested that guidelines need to be reviewed at least once every 5 years (17), and even this may be too infrequent in the case of a new innovative technology. It could also be argued that the whole process of guideline review and revision may hinder the dissemination of new knowledge. Thus, while an approach that constantly seeks the best evidence to support individual decision making will benefit the patient, better tools are needed to meet this goal, particularly in terms of the requirement for continual updating. Obviously, the clinician will value the laboratorian who is up to date and can provide the latest critically appraised evidence on the use and utility of a particular test.

Clinical Settings and Circumstances

Each patient represents a unique circumstance and there is a need to consider factors that might influence the effectiveness of a test and consequently modify the evidence base on the test's use. Issues of biological variation and comorbidities are critical in the interpretation of results; for example, as in the case of the influence of a reduction in the glomerular filtration rate on blood concentrations of NT-pro brain natriuretic peptide and homocysteine and the interpretation of drug pharmacokinetics. This aspect of EBM teaching can be the most challenging for the laboratorian as all of the relevant information may not be available. However, regular dialogue with the attending physician and regular participation in ward rounds build experience and trust between colleagues. This can be complemented by contributions to case conferences as well as audit and quality improvement exercises. Although the practice of telephoning abnormal results is primarily a service for the attending physician, this interaction can also provide valuable data on individual patient settings. However, this presupposes that non-critical or "normal results" are always of limited value (as they are not telephoned), which is clearly not the case.

Being Well Prepared

Adoption of the EBM culture, namely being able to formulate the question, search for the evidence, and provide a critically appraised summary, is the best foundation for preparedness. Undoubtedly there will be a significant degree of similarity in many clinical settings that occur; thus some common resources can be developed to reduce the burden of searching for information—and much will be committed to memory without recourse to notes or other text resources. Thus, some basic resources, e.g., reference range tables and books that list associations between abnormal results and particular diseases, can be helpful, although they do not fit into the quality framework expected of an evidence-based (laboratory) medicine approach.

Each laboratorian should find a way of accessing knowledge that suits his or her individual needs and learning style. An important part of this will be accessing knowledge resources that help to build the personal knowledge base. Many, including Sackett et al. (9) have advocated the construction of a library of critically appraised topics based on experience, that is, a logbook of clinical and laboratory experience within the framework of a critical review process.

A Multistaged Experience

As indicated earlier, the evidence-based culture is founded on formulating the question, searching for evidence, and producing a critically appraised conclusion. As experience is gained, formulating the question and accessing the best information resources become easier and searching for evidence is less onerous. The process of critical appraisal will of itself generate a number of actions and outcomes; it may help to refine the question, will identify the quality of the evidence, and help solve the problem or generate a search for evidence from other sources or through primary research. This demonstrates the iterative nature of the process and also illustrates the alternative definition that has been used for EBM—problem-based, lifelong learning. It is the continuous application of this process that underpins initial learning and maintaining of skills. Of course, many will say that this is what happens in day-to-day practice. However, as stated earlier, the process of gaining experience can be lengthy and highly variable, depending on the individual. It is well documented that expertise deteriorates with age (3). It is suggested that adopting the evidence-based culture will make the process of learning more efficient, more effective, and more lasting and help the practicing healthcare professional systematically deal with the large amount of available literature.

EDUCATIONAL OPPORTUNITIES FOR THE LABORATORIAN

It might be argued that the review of each laboratory request can provide an educational opportunity; however, frequently the quality of the information available to the laboratory may be limiting. Some of the educational opportunities are now addressed.

Telephoning Results

Virtually all laboratories have action limits for telephoning abnormal results. Typically these will be results that are indicative of life-threatening clinical crises that require immediate clinical intervention. However, this interaction can still be subjected to the "question–search–appraise–conclude" routine described earlier. These interactions are greatly appreciated by general and primary care physicians, reflecting the breadth of their clinical portfolios and their need to maintain a wide knowledge base.

Ward Rounds

Attendance at ward rounds will provide valuable experience for both the trainee and experienced laboratorian. It will give the trainee an insight into the way that clinical questions can be posed. Although time constraints may limit the benefit of this opportunity, regular attendance at ward rounds or at clinical team review meetings will provide an opportunity to review some issues arising with specific tests or for individual patients. So the main value of attending ward rounds will be to gain knowledge of context and to establish a forum for regular communication and dialogue. Finally, a collateral public relations benefit is frequently realized by visibility and interaction at ward rounds.

Case Conferences and Grand Rounds

These more formal occasions are intended as learning experiences and generally involve presentations of more unusual clinical scenarios. The intention is to broaden the experience of attendees, but the laboratorian should still employ the question–search–appraise–conclude routine in order to determine the role of laboratory medicine (18).

Clinical Audit

Often the clinical audit is primarily seen as a quality assurance tool, but it is particularly well suited to adoption of the evidence-based protocol. Although the clinical audit is a multidisciplinary team activity (chapter 11), it can also be a valuable educational tool in the laboratory. The laboratorian is constantly challenged to control the demand on the service and reduce the number of requests made. The question to ask when scrutinizing request forms should be "Why was this test requested?"

An audit of utilization can provide a valuable platform for education and continuing education of both laboratorians and users. The audit can be performed with a simple questionnaire as outlined in chapter 13. The responses typically indicate appropriate as well as inappropriate testing in terms of clinical presentation, inappropriate frequency of testing, and incorrect choice of tests. This can lead to the identification of knowledge gaps, the need for clinical protocols or clinical guidelines, the need for modification of a guideline, or the need for primary research evidence. In the context of the latter point, this raises the vexed question as to whether evidence from clinical audit projects provides a sufficiently high quality of evidence to be acceptable for incorporation onto the formulation of a guideline. Typically an audit is considered as an observational study, which is regarded as being of lower quality compared to a randomized controlled trial. Figure 2 shows a typical audit exercise of test utilization and demonstrates obvious educational benefits. Chapter 11 discusses some excellent audit exercises that provide valuable information for improvement of laboratory services.

An extension of the audit concept is represented by the development of clinical registries. These are often set up by professional bodies but also by patient advocacy organizations. Registries audit the clinical outcomes from healthcare provider organizations; many examples and details are available on the Internet (19–21)

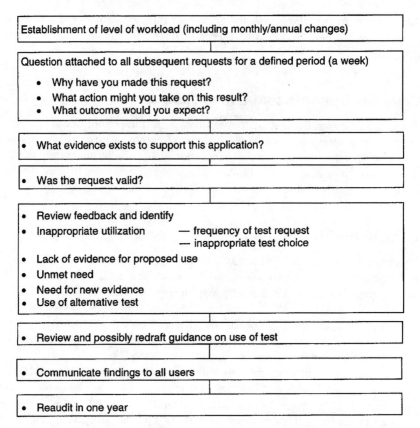

Figure 2 An example of the cycle of an audit of test utilization.

Systematic Reviews and Guidelines

A systematic review represents the basis of a clinical guideline (chapter 10). Increasingly professional organizations are setting up systematic reviews and preparing guidelines relevant to their area of expertise as part of their scientific and educational activities. Clearly guidelines enhance the position of the professional body by identifying and promoting the highest standards of practice. The rigor of this exercise is both detailed and transparent. Many guidelines are published on the Internet and are readily accessible to patients as well as health professionals.

Identifying evidence, defining quality, and clarifying deficiencies in the evidence base are crucial, and they require disciplined work (chapter 8). Such a review enables the combination of several studies and so can ensure the involvement of several teams in generating the evidence, an important factor when introducing a new test. In this way, use of a new test can be studied in several clinical settings. The review also increases confidence in the conclusions drawn from such studies.

The American Association for Clinical Chemistry has published a number of guidelines through the activity of the National Academy for Clinical Biochemistry specifically related to diagnostic tests (22, 23). These guidelines have been undertaken in collaboration with the relevant clinical physician organizations. Many clinical organizations have also established guidelines that include the use of laboratory services (24–26).

EDUCATIONAL TOOLS FOR THE LABORATORIAN

The educational tools for the laboratorian in relation to diagnostic tests can be considered in a similar way to the Sackett and Haynes discussion on the "architecture of diagnostics research" (27) and to the hierarchy of evidence required to determine the investment (or worth) in a new test as described by Fryback and Thornbury (28) and Price (29). This is illustrated in Figure 1 of chapter 2; the first level of evidence details the technical performance of the test including the impact of such issues as biological variation. The second level of evidence establishes the relationship between the test result and the disease process: the diagnostic performance. The third level shows whether the application of the test in a given situation will lead to an improved health outcome. These levels of evidence are intimately related, and it is exactly the relationship between them that defines the experience of the laboratorian in advising the clinician on a particular test result or observation on an individual patient.

One sphere in which this interrelationship is not always obvious is the influence of method imprecision and inaccuracy on a health outcome. Thus, it is important to have answers to questions like:

What is the impact of an imprecision of 15% (coefficient of variation) for a HbA1c result of 7.0% compared with an imprecision of 5%, on a diabetic's risk of developing cardiovascular disease?

What is the impact of a method with an inaccuracy of 0.5% (negative bias, actual value) for a HbA1c result of 7.0% compared to a method with no bias on a diabetic's risk of developing cardiovascular disease?

What is the impact of an inaccuracy of 1.0 ng/mL (1.0 µg/L) (negative bias) on a total prostate-specific antigen result of 4.0 ng/mL (4.0 µg/L) for a man with symptoms associated with prostatic enlargement, in terms of subsequent clinical decision making?

The first two levels of evidence are typically provided in diagnostic test compendiums (30–32). The third level is probably best achieved through systematic reviews of outcome studies involving diagnostic tests and the production of a library of critically appraised topics.

Critically Appraised Topics

There are a number of guides to the broader aspects of critical appraisal (critical appraisal tools) and one approach is described in chapter 8. The structure of a critically appraised topic as described by Sackett et al. (33) is set out in Figure 3. It comprises the clinical scenario, the three-part question as described in the educational prescription referred to earlier, the search terms, details of the study, the evidence, any commentary on the evidence and its relevance, and then the conclusions. Montori and Guyatt in chapter 1 describe an example involving the use of serum ferritin for the diagnosis of iron deficiency in a number of different patient settings.

This approach can be used to ascertain the use of a test in a specific clin-

---

Definition of clinical question

- target condition
- intervention
- outcome

Clinical scenario

Search terms

The study

- quality
- target disorder and gold standard
- patients

The evidence

- sensitivity and specificity
- predictive values
- likelihood ratios

Comments

References

Name of reviewer and date of review

Figure 3 The structure of a critically appraised topic (CAT) on the use of a diagnostic test.

ical setting or the use of a testing modality, e.g., POCT. An example for the use of POCT for HbA1c performed at the time of the clinic visit is illustrated in Figure 4. A second example on the potential use of brain (B-type) natriuretic peptide to guide therapy in patients with heart failure is illustrated in Figure 5.

Experience shows that one of the key features of producing a critically appraised topic is the search strategy that is used. As detailed in chapter 6,

---

Clinical question: Will the availability of the HbA1c result at the time of the clinic visit lead to improved longer term glycemic control?

Clinical scenario   — diabetes mellitus
                               — POCT during clinic visit HbA1c
                               — Improved glycemic control (judged by reduction of HbA1c)

Search terms: HbA1c, point-of-care testing, diabetes mellitus

The study   — randomized controlled trial
                       — laboratory HbA1c measurement at 6 and 12 months
                       — 186 type 1 diabetics

The evidence: HbA1c fell at 6 and 12 months, −0.57% and −0.40%, p<0.01 in POCT group, only −0.11% and 0.195 in control group, not significant, all compared with baseline. No difference in rates of hypoglycemic events.

Comments: a similar study question was addressed in another study where POCT testing for HbA1c was compared with conventional laboratory testing for HbA1c in an observational study of two neighboring hospital clinic procedures with similar findings, i.e., POCT delivery of HbA1c led to lower levels being achieved.

References
1. Cagliero E, Levina E, Nathan D. Immediate feedback of HbA1c levels improves glycemic control in type 1 and insulin-treated type 2 diabetic patients. Diabetes Care 1999;22:1785–9.
2. Grieve R, Beech R, Vincent J, Mazurkiewicz J. Near patient testing in diabetes clinics: appraising the costs and outcomes. Health Technol Assoc 1999;3:1–74.

Name of reviewer and date of review:

C. P. Price   December 15, 2000

Figure 4 An example of a critically appraised topic (CAT) dealing with an operational issue.

Clinical question: Will BNP guided treatment be more effective than current clinical practice in patients with heart failure?

Clinical scenario   — patient newly diagnosed with heart failure
— primary or secondary care setting
— commenced on treatment with angiotensin-converting enzyme inhibitor

Search terms: brain natriuretic peptide, heart failure, treatment

The study: patients were randomized to receive treatment guided by either brain natriuretic peptide level or standardized clinical assessment

The evidence: during follow-up for at least 6 months the cardiac events in the BNP guided group were lower (19 vs 54, p=0.02) than the control group. A total of 27% of the BNP group compared with 53% of the control group experienced events, p=0.034

Comments: there were only 69 patients in the study. A recent review while stating that more data were needed indicated that, taken with other data, this indicated that BNP guided therapy might be helpful to both clinician and patient.

References
1. Troughton RW, Frampton CM, Yandle TG, Espiner EA, Nicholls MG, Richards AM. Treatment of heart failure guided by plasma aminoterminal brain natriuretic peptide (N-BNP) concentrations. Lancet 2000;355:1126–30.
2. Cowie MR, Mendez GF. BNP and congestive heart failure. Progr Cardio Dis 2001; 44: 293-321.

Name of reviewer and date of review:

R.H. Christenson   February 18, 2003

Figure 5 An example of a critically appraised topic (CAT) dealing with an issue of clinical test utility.

too broad a search will generate a large number of largely irrelevant papers, while a highly focused strategy may miss the few key papers.

RESOURCES FOR TEACHING EVIDENCE-BASED LABORATORY MEDICINE

Many resources have been described in this book that will help readers gain more experience in the practice of evidence-based (laboratory) medicine and disseminate the culture to others. A search on the Internet using the term "evidence based medicine" yielded more than 1.3 million hits (on April 6, 2003). A search using the term "evidence based laboratory medicine" yielded no sites, but the term "evidence base diagnostics" yielded 122,000 sites. Some of these resources are set out below with a brief summary of contents and some observations on their practical utility.

www.aacc.org/ebm describes the EBM Resource Centre for the American Association of Clinical Chemistry. The site lists some key published papers on evidence-based laboratory medicine as well as leading EBM journals. It lists the articles dealing with evidence on diagnostic tests published in *Clinical Chemistry* (which numbered a total of 305 on the day accessed, April 6, 2003). There are links to government EBM-related sites in the United States and the United Kingdom as well as a number of important private EBM sites. The Association works closely with the Agency for Healthcare Research and Quality to identify topics that should be considered by the Agency for systematic review; the site invites readers to submit proposals.

www.bmj.com/cgi/collection/diagnostic_tests is a collection of papers published on diagnostic tests in the *British Medical Journal* with links to related articles in other journals.

www.cebm.utoronto.ca is the site for the Centre for Evidence-Based Medicine. The goal of the site is to "help develop, disseminate, and evaluate resources that can be used to practice and teach EBM for undergraduate, postgraduate and continuing education for health care professionals from a variety of clinical disciplines." The site is also used to support the book by Sackett et al. referenced on occasions during this chapter (9, 13, 33). In addition to complementing this excellent book, it provides useful teaching materials, a critical appraisal worksheet, a glossary of terms, a comprehensive list of EBM resources, and links to other EBM sites.

www.cche.net/principles/content_all.asp hosts the User's Guide to the Medical Literature produced by the *Journal of the American Medical Association*. The goal is to "package, disseminate, and present health knowledge in ways that facilitate its optimum use." Visitors are alerted to significant EBM resources as they become available, and structured abstracts are provided that identify the quality of the information and its applicability.

www.clinicalevidence.org is a compendium of evidence on the effects of common clinical interventions. It provides a concise account of the state of knowledge, based on thorough searches of the literature.

www.ebm.bmjjournals.com is the site associated with the journal *Evidence-Based Medicine*. The journal specializes in taking reviews from the literature and providing a succinct critique of the review and its applicability to routine practice. There is a section on diagnostic tools.

www.cebm.jr2.ox.ac.uk is the site for the Centre of Evidence-Based Medicine in Oxford. The website includes an EBM Toolbox with various tools for practicing and teaching EBM. It includes the CATMaker, which is a software program for the user to create a 1-page summary of evidence.

www.cochrane.org is the base site for the Cochrane Collaboration. This includes the Cochrane Library, which provides high quality evidence through systematic reviews performed to a high standard. It also includes a register of controlled trials, a list of resources for reviewing evidence, and a list of upcoming EBM-related Cochrane events.

www.healthlinks.washington.edu/clinical/guidelines.html is a University of Washington site that includes useful information resources including much of that referenced in this chapter including Patient Orientated Evidence that Matters (POEMS).

www.healthweb.org is a site associated with the Library of Health Sciences of the University of Illinois at Chicago. It contains a useful guide to searching the literature.

www.jr2.ox.ac.uk/bandolier/booths/booths/diag.html is the Bandolier site specifically associated with diagnostics. The Bandolier site is well worth a visit because it provides a broader perspective. This diagnostics site alludes to the dearth of good evidence on diagnostic test performance but includes some good examples that provide useful guidance on what is required to yield good evidence.

www.nelh.nhs.uk/diagnosis.asp is the site of the National Electronic Library of Health, which discusses examples of good evidence on diagnostic tests.

www.poems.msu.edu/Infomastery is a site associated with Michigan State University that incorporates a useful web-based course on critical appraisal of the medical literature.

www.shef.ac.uk/~scharr/ir/netting/first.html is a website that claims to provide a complete list of evidence-based practice resources available on the Internet. There are more than 140 listings providing some very valuable material.

www.tripdatabase.com provides direct hyperlinked access to the largest collection of evidence-based material on the web by searching more than 75 sites for high-quality information. This includes articles from some of the major on-line medical journals.

www.ucl.ac.uk/openlearning/uebpp/uebpp.htm is the site associated with the Department of Primary Care and Population Sciences at University College, London. It provides information on a number of useful resources for EBM training.

http://www.ckchl-mb.nl/ifcc/index.htm is the International Federation for Clinical Chemistry's EBM website. The purpose of this website is to enhance the understanding, use, and performance of systematic reviews and to facilitate rational laboratory utilization. The site stresses interdisciplinary involvement with clinicians and has numerous useful references, particularly on meta-analysis and systematic reviews.

www.york.ac.uk/inst/crd/welcome.htm is the site for the NHS Centre for Reviews and Dissemination and is related to the U.K. Cochrane Centre. The goal of the Centre is to produce reviews concerning the clinical and cost effectiveness of healthcare interventions. It provides access to several databases including a database of structured abstracts of good quality systematic reviews (DARE); these reviews comment on methodological features of reviews and summarize the author's conclusions.

http://tudor.szote.u-szeged.hu/webeng/be_e.php is an EBM site with versions in both Hungarian and English that was developed in collaboration with a grant from British government. A stated purpose of the site is to promote scientific medicine in a way that is enjoyable to the user. The site is easily navigated and is organized based on: (1) Resources, (2) Activities, and (3) Know How Needed. In particular, the teaching aids listed on the home page is a rich source of EBM teaching information and material.

SUMMARY

Teaching evidence-based (laboratory) medicine begins with gaining experience of the process for accurately defining the question, finding the evidence, and then critically appraising the evidence to convey the key message that summarizes the utility of the test. This process should be patient focused and become part of the routine practice at the interface between the laboratorian and the clinical user of the laboratory service. Laboratorians should strive to make this process part of the accepted culture of their everyday clinical interaction and organization.

There are abundant opportunities for adopting this approach to practice and a number of vehicles for disseminating this culture, as well as the product of this philosophy. There are still challenges to making this an efficient and practical routine feature of daily professional life. These include the ability to define exactly the relevant question, to develop an efficient approach to searching for and reviewing the evidence, and then making the output readily available to all healthcare professionals who might use it.

REFERENCES

1. Sackett DL, Rosenberg WMC, Gray JAM, Haynes RB, Richardson WS. Evidence-based medicine: what it is and what it isn't. Br Med J 1996;312:71–2.
2. Dawes M, Davies P, Gray A, Mant J, Seers K, Snowball, eds. Evidence-Based Practice; a primer for health care professionals. Churchill Livingstone, Edinburgh, 2001:1–254.
3. Ramsey PG, Carline JD, Inui TS, Larson EB, LoGerfo JP, Norcini JJ, et al. Changes over time in the knowledge base of internists. J Am Med Assoc 1991;266:1103–7.
4. Thomas P. Competence, revalidation and continuing professional development—a business package. Ann R Coll Surg Engl 1999;81:13–5.
5. Bonini P, Plebani M, Ceriotti F, Rubboli F. Errors in laboratory medicine. Clin Chem 2002;48:691–8.
6. Plebani M, Carraro P. Mistakes in a stat laboratory: types and frequency. Clin Chem 1997;43:1348–51.
7. Kilpatrick ES, Holding S. Use of computer terminals on wards to access emergency test results: a retrospective audit. Br Med J 2001;322:1101–3.
8. Price CP, Barnes IC. Laboratory medicine in the United Kingdom: 1948–1998 and beyond. Clin Chim Acta 2000;290:5–36.
9. Sackett DL, Straus SE, Richardson WS, Rosenberg W, Haynes RB. Teaching methods. In: Evidence-based medicine. how to practice and teach EBM, 2nd ed. Edinburgh: Churchill Livingstone, 2000:183–218.
10. Guyatt G, Haynes B, Jaeschke R, Cook D, Greenhalgh T, Meade M, et al. Introduction: the philosophy of evidence-based medicine. In: Guyatt G, Rennie D, eds. User's guide to the medical literature. A manual for evidence-based clinical practice. Chicago: J Am Med Assoc and Archive Journals, American Medical Association, 2002:3–12.
11. www.labtestsonline.org
12. Price CP. Evidence-based laboratory medicine. Ned Tijdschr Klin Chem 2001;26:236–42.
13. Price CP. Point of care testing: potential for tracking disease management outcomes. Dis Manage Health Outcomes 2002;10:749–61.
14. Sackett DL, Straus SE, Richardson WS, Rosenberg W, Haynes RB. Asking answerable clinical questions. In: Evidence-based medicine. How to practice and teach EBM, 2nd ed. Edinburgh: Churchill Livingstone, 2000:13–27.
15. Richardson WS, Wilson MC, Nishikawa J, Hayward RSA. The well built clinical question: a key to evidence-based decisions. ACP J Club 1995;123:A12–3.
16. Richardson WS, Burdette SD. Practice corner: taking evidence in hand. Evidence-based medicine 2003;8:4–5.

17. Shekelle PG, Ortiz E, Rhodes S, Morton SC Eccles MP, Grimshaw JM, et al. Validity of the Agency for Healthcare Research and Quality clinical practice guidelines: how quickly do guidelines become outdated? J Am Med Assoc 2001;286:1461–7.
18. Freedman DB, Hooper J, Wood PJ, Worthington DJ, Price CP, eds. Challenges at the clinical interface: case histories for clinical biochemists. Washington DC: AACC Press, 2001:1–252.
19. European Network of Cancer Registries at http://www.encr.com.fr (accessed on April 10, 2003).
20. Gaucher Registry at http://www.gaucherregistry.com (accessed on April 10, 2003).
21. Cystic Fibrosis Registry of Australia at http://www.cysticfibrosisaustralia. org/dataregistry.shtml (accessed on April 10, 2003).
22. Sacks DB, Bruns DE, Goldstein DE, Maclaren NK, McDonald JM, Parrott M. Guidelines and recommendations for laboratory analysis in the diagnosis and management of diabetes mellitus. Clin Chem 2002;48:436–72.
23. Dufour DR, Lott JA, Nolte FS, Gretch JA, Koff RS, Seeff LB. Diagnosis and monitoring of hepatic injury. II. Recommendations for use of laboratory tests in screening, diagnosis, and monitoring. Clin Chem 2000;46:2050–68.
24. National Kidney Foundation K/DOQI Clinical practice guidelines for chronic kidney disease; evaluation, classification and stratification at http://www. kidney.org/professional/doqi/kdoqi/p1_exec.htm (accessed on April 10, 2003).
25. American Association of Clinical Endocrinology. Medical guidelines for clinical practice for the evaluation and treatment of hyperthyroidism and hypothyroidism at http://www.aace.com/clin/guidelines/hypo_hyper.pdf (accessed on April 10, 2003).
26. National Institute of Health. Consensus statement on osteoporosis, prevention, diagnosis and treatment at http://odp.od.nih.gov/consensus/con/111/111_intro. htm (accessed on April 10, 2003).
27. Sackett DL, Haynes RB, The architecture of diagnostic research. Br Med J 2002;321:539–41.
28. Fryback FG, Thornbury JR. The efficacy of diagnostic imaging. Med Decis Making 1991;11:88–94.
29. Price CP. Evidence-based laboratory medicine: supporting decision-making. Clin Chem 2000;46:1041–50.
30. Tietz NW, ed. Clinical guide to laboratory tests. Philadelphia: Saunders, 1990:1–931.
31. Wallach J. Interpretation of diagnostic tests: a synopsis of laboratory medicine, 5th ed. Boston: Little, Brown, 1992:1–933.
32. Jacobs DS, Kasten BL, DeMott WR, Wolfson WL. Laboratory test handbook. Cleveland: Lexi-Comp/Mosby, 1988:1–921.
33. Sackett DL, Straus SE, Richardson WS, Rosenberg W, Haynes RB. Diagnosis and screening. In: Evidence-based medicine. How to practice and teach EBM, 2nd ed. Edinburgh: Churchill Livingstone, 2000:63–93.

13

Adopting the Principles of Evidence-Based Laboratory Medicine in Routine Practice

Christopher P. Price and Robert H. Christenson

It is impossible to decry the philosophy and fundamental principles of evidence-based medicine (1) and yet its inherent simplicity is sometimes contradicted by its apparent success to date and the criticism that it engenders in its application (2, 3). The confusion arises in part because of the complex nature of the whole clinical process, the amount of information available with which to make decisions, and the variability of human interaction (4, 5). Guyatt et al. (6) stated that there are two fundamental principles of evidence-based medicine. First, in clinical decision making, the evidence has to be balanced by the benefits and risks, inconvenience, and cost of alternative strategies, and second there is an hierarchy of evidence. This immediately places the decision-maker in a position of having to collect several pieces of information and then make a balanced judgment that is appropriate to that situation. Clearly, the greater the reliability of the information, the greater the confidence of the decision-maker, and the better the outcome. Evidence-based medicine has also been described as a process of problem-based, continuous lifelong learning which also highlights the importance of keeping up to date and of good communication.

THINGS TO CONSIDER

The reliability of information on the utility of a diagnostic test depends on the quality of the analytical performance of the test(s) being used at the time of the consultation, the quality of the evidence that has been developed on the clinical utility of that test, and the relevance or appropriateness of that evidence to the clinical setting of the current consultation (7). The efficacy of the test depends on the assimilation of all of these pieces of information, and the correct decision being made in light of all of the information available, together with the correct action being implemented. The efficacy will be demonstrated in the quality of the health outcome. Unfortunately, all peer-reviewed literature is not created equal. Yet there is a tendency to lump papers together and then accept them as representing the truth because they appear in a peer-reviewed journal. Several chapters in this book have highlighted the important issues that must be considered when designing robust diagnostic accuracy and outcome studies and the procedures for reviewing and reporting data. Good quality data are the cornerstone of the information that generates the knowledge that informs practice.

The health outcome from any clinical decision and intervention can be broadly viewed in clinical and economic terms. As illustrated earlier in this book (chapter 4), the clinical outcome is seen ultimately in improved morbidity and mortality. Additional indicators of improved clinical outcome include improved mobility and reduced disability as well as improved patient satisfaction. Economic outcomes can be viewed in the context of the costs of care set against the benefit to the patient or more widely to society (8). This overview clearly shows that the collection of improved outcomes data accruing from the use of a diagnostic test is both challenging and involves considerable complexity in its elaboration (9, 10). However, the confidence that is gained from having robust evidence available cannot be denied. The challenges associated with demonstrating improved outcomes partly relate to the difficulty of mimicking the consultation process in such a way that a valid experiment can be conducted without introducing bias to the final result. This is not dissimilar from routine practice with the need to have complete compliance with the clinical protocol for that unique situation in order for the expected outcome to be delivered. Thus, if the result is not accessed by the clinician, then the outcome will not be attained if the test was important to the decision making (11).

Some examples of different clinical scenarios in which a diagnostic test can be involved are shown in Figure 1; this description is still an oversimplification of the multifaceted process involved in the diagnosis and management of disease. It is clear that there has to be compliance with test, decision, and intervention in order to obtain the outcome. While there is considerable debate on the best study design to demonstrate the clinical utility of a diagnostic test (12, 13), there have been few studies in which the patients have been randomized to receive the test result and thereby demonstrating, in an unequivocal way, the role of the test result in decision making.

Sackett et al. (14) in a book on clinical epidemiology, subtitled "a basic science for clinical medicine", in describing the clinical examination, pointed out the opportunity for clinical disagreement and the ways in which

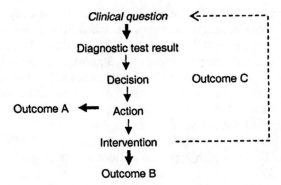

Figure 1 The three main classes of decision cascade that involve a diagnostic test where outcome A is a test result used to rule out an action and/or a diagnosis, outcome B is a test result used to rule in an action and/or a diagnosis, and outcome C is a test to inform a decision and an action that has to be repeated at a given frequency to deliver the desired outcome.

this variation could be minimized. They described the construction of diagnostic hypotheses and capturing clinical data to resolve these hypotheses. The use of a diagnostic test provides a means of resolving these hypotheses. These same authors also pointed out that, while the term "diagnosis" is used, the same kind of decision making is applied to predicting the subsequent course of the disease, to predicting the response to an intervention, and to assessing the actual effect of the intervention. Thus, when a test is being considered, the clinician has a question for which it is hoped that the result will provide an answer (7, 15, and chapter 2). There should then follow some form of decision, an action being initiated, all leading to an improved outcome. The collection of clinical data from observation and clinical examination in the first instance helps to formulate the question, and the quality of the evidence on a test helps to decide whether the result is helpful in obtaining an answer.

The complexity of demonstrating an association between the diagnostic test and a health outcome is compounded by the evidence that the quality of studies on diagnostic accuracy and health outcomes is poor and several systematic reviews have pointed to the dearth of good quality evidence (16–18). Thus, Hobbs et al. (19), in a systematic review of the use of point-of-care testing in primary care, showed that less than 10% of the papers identified by a comprehensive search met the basic quality criteria, and, in those that did, very few focused on the demonstration of a clinical outcome from the use of this testing modality. Balk et al. (20) in a review of cardiac markers found that few of the papers focused on how the measurements of biochemical markers aided decision making and therefore could be seen to improve the health outcome. Other investigators pointed to the need for more evidence in situations where practice is seen to be well established, albeit not necessarily founded on the highest quality of evidence (21). This can cause considerable problems when long-established practice is called into question, as it would probably be considered unethical to embark on a randomized controlled trial of a diagnostic test as it would involve denying a test result to someone who would previously have had access to that result. In most of these instances, the investigators have not focused on the clinical questions being asked and therefore have not set up the right study or monitored the relevant outcomes. In this situation, the only way forward is to perform some form of audit, which is effectively an observational study and carries with it certain criticisms with respect to the quality of the results (22).

Sackett and Haynes (23) described the "architecture of diagnostics research" in a way that illustrated the logic of studies on diagnostic performance, highlighting the importance of interpretation of data, correct study design, and protocol compliance. They described four phases of research into diagnostic performance as:

- **Phase 1:** establishing whether the results in the target disorder (the disease in which the test is to be applied) are different from those in normal individuals
- **Phase 2:** whether patients with certain results (e.g., elevated levels compared with "normals") are more likely to have the target disease compared with others
- **Phase 3:** whether the test result distinguishes between those who have the disease and those who do not in a population of individuals in whom the disease is suspected (e.g., those who are "at risk")
- **Phase 4:** whether those who have the test (and who need the test) enjoy a better health outcome compared to those who do not have access to (but need) the test

They then went on to show with the aid of the data on likelihood ratios derived from published studies how the diagnostic performance of the test will be influenced by the patients selected for study and by the study design. In what they described as a phase 1 study, brain (B-type) natriuretic peptide (BNP) levels are clearly elevated in patients diagnosed with heart failure. They showed from a phase 2 study that BNP looked promising as both a "rule in" and a "rule out" test (likelihood ratios of 13 and 0.03, respectively). However, when they moved to a phase 3 study in which the test was used to "identify" those patients considered to be at risk of developing heart failure into those with and without evidence of heart failure (defined by use of the gold standard diagnostic test), the performance of the test was not so encouraging (likelihood ratios of 1.3 and 0.4, respectively). In this phase 3 study, the clinical question and setting are getting much closer to the way in which the test might be used, therefore focusing more accurately on the clinical application. The phase 4 study focuses on the integration of the test into the decision-making process and compliance with that process, which is where the randomized controlled trial provides the most robust experimental design. Critically, it is in this latter phase of this diagnostic architecture or study design that the availability of the diagnostic test result has become the rate-limiting step and therefore in which its role can be truly judged.

Fryback and Thornbury (24) described the evidence that was required in order to make a decision to introduce a new test, and others have supported its use in both clinical and operational decision making (25, 26). The cascade of evidence is illustrated in the left portion of Figure 2. The core of this portfolio lies in the technical and diagnostic performance of the test, supported by the outcomes data to indicate that the expectation of the test is then met when applied to practice. However, the availability of evidence will not guarantee benefit as there is the need to ensure that there is proper dissemination of the information on the performance of the test, education of users, funding to ensure the test can be delivered, and compliance in practice. Thus, evidence on the utility of a test, the core of evidence-based laboratory medicine (EBLM), plays a central role in the implementation and maintenance of a high-quality service (Figure 3).

WHY IS EBLM IMPORTANT TODAY?

While it is the goal of all laboratory professionals to deliver the highest quality of service, there are many challenges to that aspiration:

- Increasing workloads
- New technology being constantly introduced

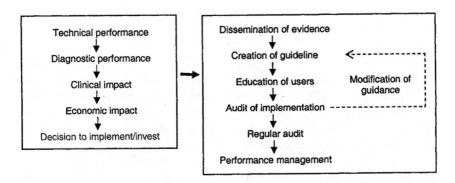

Figure 2 The portfolio of evidence that should be used to support reimbursement for/investment in a diagnostic test (left-hand box) and the activities required to ensure effective implementation when the evidence favors investment (right-hand box).

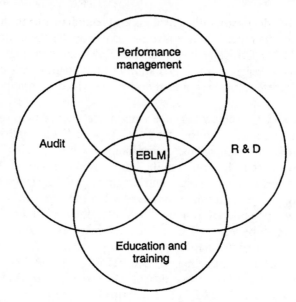

Figure 3 Research and development, continuing education, audit, and performance management are the core of the application of evidence-based practice in delivering a high-quality service.

- Demand seen as uncontrollable
- Claims of too much unnecessary testing
- Limited perceived role in outcomes
- Seen as commoditized, low value
- Heavy burden of scientific literature
- Transition of evidence to practice is slow
- Continuing education is poor
- Investment in diagnostics is flawed (cost not benefit)

There is a continuous stream of new tests being described and new technology developed, which adds to the ever-increasing workload seen in most laboratories. There is also perceived to be an inability to control the demand (27) while little attention is paid to the impact that the test result has on the health outcome. This has led to the call for an outcomes agenda for laboratory medicine to help answer some of the questions raised (28, 29).

Implementation of new diagnostic tests, in common with interventions (30), is slow. This may be due to problems of continuing education and the difficulties associated with changing practice (31), as well as the problems associated with gaining funding (reimbursement) for new tests. All of these issues are obviously compounded by the poor quality of evidence on the utility of new tests, the inability to demonstrate improved health outcomes, and the delays in bringing data into the peer-reviewed literature.

While the philosophy and culture of EBLM plays a key role in the day-to-day practice of medicine as well as the implementation of new technologies, it is important to recognize where EBLM can be a valuable practical tool in the definition, implementation, and maintenance of a high-quality service. How can evidence be used in day-to-day practice?

QUALITY OF SERVICE

The "service need" defines the applied research agenda that drives the search for the evidence of effectiveness associated with any test or intervention. The identification of need will then help to formulate the specific clinical question(s) that help to map out the study design to elicit the evidence on effectiveness. The study design will itself reflect the way in which the test is going to be used as part of the clinical consultation that constitutes the interaction between the patient and the clinician. The surrogate markers used in the design of many studies involving diagnostic tests are often the markers that are used in routine clinical practice for disease management, as well as indices for performance management; examples include HbA1c in diabetes mellitus, cholesterol in cardiovascular disease, and hepatitis C antigen testing in liver disease. The results from such studies will define the expectations of the test process and help to quantify the outcome. This effectively establishes the standard or the benchmark for that "clinical process or episode" and from which the quality of service can be defined and measured.

Exercise 1: What are the most likely clinical questions being asked, and in what clinical settings, when requesting any of the following tests: troponin I, C-reactive protein, brain (B-type) natriuretic peptide, cystatin C, or urine albumin:creatinine ratio?

Exercise 2: What will the requester do with the result? What decision might be made and what action taken?

As has been pointed out earlier, the translation of evidence into practice requires a thorough process of education and dissemination of results. The form of the original evidence can often be modified into some form of guideline or algorithm which is then tested in randomized trial or, more commonly, in the initial wave of application of the test. A review of practice may then lead to a modification of the guidelines followed by further education and dissemination. In this way, a guideline can be validated (7) and the strength of the evidence enhanced by the inclusion of a larger population of data. This step, in addition, will identify any opportunities for generalizability of the data to populations of patients beyond that of the original studies.

Thus, the principles of EBLM are central to establishing the quality of practice (Figure 3).

GUIDELINES

The establishment of clinical guidelines is seen as an important element of initiatives to enhance the quality of patient care (32). It is a way of systematizing care pathways, which at the outset enables the researcher to identify all of the relevant research questions and the potential outcomes. This is undoubtedly true in the case of diagnostic tests where there remain many contentious issues concerning the way in which tests are used, for example, in the frequency of testing. Some examples are:

- Optimal frequency of blood glucose testing in diabetes
- Optimal frequency of HbA1c testing in diabetes management
- Accuracy and precision of glucose test for diabetes management
- Accuracy and precision of PSA test for "rule in/rule out" of prostate cancer
- Preferred tests for assessment of liver dysfunction
- Frequency of testing of liver dysfunction
- Preferred tests for monitoring thyroid hormone replacement

The establishment of a guideline also provides the spur to review the data on the utility of a test or an intervention, the particular way in which it may be used, as well as the benefit that derives from its use. The holistic nature of a guideline also helps to identify the way in which practice may need to change when implementing a new test or intervention. There are several examples in the literature, for example, with point-of-care testing, where a change has not generated the expected benefits, which in retrospect has been thought to be due to the absence of the change in practice needed to achieve the benefit. A guideline also provides an overview of the quality of the evidence which indicates the robustness of the data on effectiveness of a test and also how wide the applicability of the test might be in different clinical settings (33). Much of the material for a guideline will have been generated from a systematic review of the peer-reviewed literature (chapter 8). However, the guideline does allow the potential application which is unsupported by adequate evidence to be highlighted.

Exercise 3: What evidence is there to support the validity of the clinical questions that you formulated in Exercise 1, or what evidence would you want to see?

The guideline provides the foundation for the education of users of a service as well as providing the benchmark against which to audit the successful implementation of a service. Thus, the guideline becomes the platform for maintaining good clinical governance (34). However, the use of guidelines to change practice is very challenging and many barriers to change have been identified (35, 36). Roe et al. (37) recently reviewed the use of guidelines in the management of patients with acute coronary syndromes. They described the underuse of evidence-based therapies, setting out the strategies to overcome the challenges facing quality improvement, as well as reviewing specific initiatives to improve the care of patients with non ST-segment elevation acute coronary syndromes.

Exercise 4: What clinical outcomes would you expect to find, and what measures would you use, to support your claims for the clinical questions and settings that you identified in Exercise 1?

AUDIT

While audit has attracted a particular connotation in the context of healthcare (clinical audit), the term has a broader meaning and can be used to describe a number of activities under the broad umbrella of "official auditing of accounts" *(Oxford English Dictionary)*. Thus, clinical audit can be described as the review of cases against the benchmark of current best practice (38, chapter 10); the wider application can be used to describe benchmarking of performance against peers and regular review of practice against established performance. All three are valid tools as part of an ongoing quality improvement program and as part of a performance management program.

Laboratory Audit

In the case of the laboratory, the audit can take the form of a review of the way in which a test is used. This may be stimulated by a rapid rise in the number of tests requested or a failure to meet targets for defined outcome measures. Typically, workload increases are associated with either an increasing awareness of a particular test or disease (e.g., prostate-specific antigen and its claimed use in screening for prostate cancer and C-reactive protein in acute coronary syndromes) or the publication of a number of articles in respected clinical journals. The approach to such an audit will begin with a review of the workload trends over the past months and comparison with related indicators of clinical activity, e.g., admissions and clinic visits.

It is then necessary to determine the reason for the increased level of requesting from the service users. One of the most effective ways of doing this is to require an additional piece of information to be provided when a request is made. A question can be posed in a number of ways; some examples are:

- What clinical question were you asking?
- What are the clinical indications for this test request?
- Why do you require this result urgently?
- What decision would you make on receipt of this test result?
- What action would you take on receipt of this test result?
- What are the risks associated with not having a test result?
- What is the expected outcome from having this test result?
- What is the evidence for the utility of this test?

This approach is most effective when electronic requesting is available because it is possible to ensure a high level of compliance with the enquiry, as the test request can be blocked until the additional question is answered! A paper-based exercise is unlikely to achieve such a high level of compliance.

Exercise 5: What questions would you formulate to find the reason for a large increase in the workload of any of the markers identified in Exercise 1?

The responses can then be used to identify the clinical questions being asked and these can be matched against the evidence for the clinical utility of the test. This approach can identify misconceptions about the utility of the test and resolve confusion with other tests as well as address abuse of the service! The exercise will help to identify clinical needs (unanswered clinical questions), disseminate the evidence of utility in the situations identified, and identify misconceptions and ignorance on the use of test results. It provides a vehicle for education and updating of knowledge on the service. It may also identify new needs for which the evidence of clinical utility has not been generated, creating a forward-looking research agenda.

However, perhaps of greatest importance, audit provides an opportunity to demonstrate an ongoing approach to demand management that is closely linked with problem-based, continuous service improvement. This can then be linked into a more holistic approach to performance management, because there is a greater appreciation of the role that the diagnostic test plays in the whole process of disease management.

Benchmarking and Performance Indicators

An important management tool in the modern health service, which focuses on both clinical and economic outcomes, is benchmarking (39). This is now an established part of management practice and which operates at a number of levels of perspective. It may operate within the laboratory, comparing this year's performance with that of last year; it may operate as an interlaboratory exercise or at the other extreme it may operate at a national or international level where high level clinical and economic indicators are employed, e.g., morbidity and mortality figures.

Many of the audits and benchmarking activities associated with laboratory services to date have focused on workload, staff, equipment, and space productivity (40). Generally, these are easily measured parameters which may be regarded as "indicators of process efficiency" (41); however, they do not provide any information on the effectiveness of the service. In order to gain an insight into the effectiveness of a service, it is necessary to identify performance indicators that will reflect the way in which the laboratory medicine service is being used (42). This requires an identical approach to the study of the clinical process that is used when designing an outcomes study and invariably will use many of the surrogate outcomes markers that will have been used in such a study.

This is not an easy task and the complexity is illustrated in the example shown in Figure 4. Furthermore, it is no easy task to conduct such an audit when many of the indicators will not be available. However, it would be difficult to rebut this approach as providing a more valid means of studying the effectiveness of the laboratory medicine service.

Exercise 6: What performance indicators would you chose to demonstrate the efficacy of the laboratory service for the markers identified in Exercise 1?

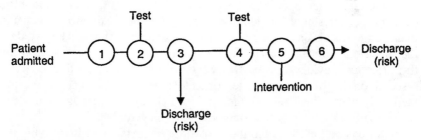

Figure 4 Some of the key decision points in the case of a patient admitted with chest pain, and the performance indicators that might be used to assess the effectiveness of the laboratory service (1) triage strategy for patients admitted with chest pain, (2) access to a rapid troponin measurement service, (3) algorithm for rule out of acute coronary syndrome including assessment of risk of further cardiac event, (4) further test to rule in or rule out acute coronary syndrome, (5) thrombolytic, platelet aggregation inhibitor therapy, or mechanical intervention, and (6) assessment of cardiac risk before discharge. Performance indicators can be built onto these decision points and could include speed of troponin service, length of stay in admissions unit, "time to needle," total length of stay, and morbidity and mortality indices.

The most holistic approach to audit that identifies with the patient, the provider, and the societal perspective is demonstrated by the disease-specific registries that have been set up in many countries and the observational studies that they perform. Thus, the National Registry for Myocardial Infarction has been in operation since 1990 and collects data from more than 1600 hospitals on the practices and outcomes associated with patients suffering from acute coronary syndromes. One of the key objectives is to evaluate treatment procedures and monitor outcomes (43). The U.K. Renal Registry describes its work as "facilitating comparative audit by means of a carefully defined data set." It collects indicators of the quality of care and audits against recommended standards with the goal of improved care (44). The Finnish Diabetes Register is another example that describes its role in quality control and the assessment of care (45). All of these initiatives are founded on standards of practice informed by good quality outcomes evidence, and the observational studies help to enhance the quality of the standards.

ECONOMICS AND BUSINESS CASES

While the approach to funding of diagnostic services differs throughout the world, there is an underlying need to understand the costs associated with the provision of such services and the financial benefits that will accrue from these services. This is the essence of health economics (chapter 9). It is clear from the foregoing discussion that this is a complex subject (46) and it has been called an inexact science. However, the essence of health economics is to understand the balance between cost and benefit, and therefore the question becomes how can health economic data be used in the policy and management decision making of laboratory medicine. If one acknowledges that decisions about the care of patients or populations are based on the three factors of evidence, values, and resources (47), then the final phase of research on diagnostic tests as described by Sackett and Haynes (23) is immediately placed high on the agenda of all policy and management decision-makers, in the context of outcomes, not merely costs.

All texts on health economics stress the importance of identifying the context of the analysis together with other quality criteria (48), and a review of papers on health economic analyses has shown how infrequently all of these criteria are met (49). In the field of laboratory medicine, the majority of papers focus on the "cost per test," which is an extremely narrow perspective and will only allow a comparison of different ways of delivering a service as long the outcomes are identical. Many of the early papers on point-of-care testing focused on cost per test, ignoring the fact that the potential outcomes from these two testing modalities could be quite different. A good example here would be the benefit of frequent home glucose monitoring in gestational diabetes, rather than having to depend on an infrequent laboratory delivered service (50, 51). At the other extreme, the economic analyses associated with the Diabetes Control and Complications Trial (52) and the United Kingdom Prospective Diabetes Study (53) have both shown that there is an economic benefit to more intensive management of diabetes by a reduction in the costs of managing the complications (54).

How can this thinking be applied in laboratory medicine? It is obvious that there needs to be some form of analysis of process efficiency from an economic perspective. However, while stating the obvious, it is important to stress that the benefit from the laboratory service will always be found outside the laboratory. This is where the perspective is important in terms of the economic analysis being conducted in the context of the decision-making environment. A test result may therefore bring value to the immediate clinical team using the result, to the local healthcare provider (physician office/health center, hospital), to the local payer (Health Management Organization or Insurer in the United States), Primary Care Trust (in the United Kingdom), to the government, or to society as a whole.

In the United States and other countries where there is reimbursement for diagnostic procedures, the economic case will be made in tandem with the evidence of clinical effectiveness and in the context of improved morbidity and mortality. In the United Kingdom and other countries where there is central funding for healthcare, the case often has to be made at a more local level. However, the underlying case will be common to both decision-making scenarios; the case for investment in the test should be made in the context of the improved and economic outcomes.

Some economic benefits that might be highlighted in making such a case are associated with a reduction in:

- Test utilization
- Time to decision
- Pharmaceutical utilization
- Blood product utilization
- "Clinical" staffing requirement
- Space requirement
- Length of stay
- Cost per episode

A review of these potential benefits shows that, in many cases, the delivery of the test has to be accompanied by a change in practice in order to deliver the benefit; this is invariably the case when instituting a point-of-care testing strategy.

There are several examples in the literature where evidence of improved clinical outcomes can then be used to model a change in practice that will deliver improved clinical and economic benefits; many of these focus on the reduced utilization of hospital resources (55–57).

Exercise 7: Construct a business case for the reimbursement/investment in the markers identified in Exercise 1, identifying the potential clinical and economic benefits from using the tests.

CHANGE MANAGEMENT

The foregoing discussion has illustrated the potential power of good quality evidence to deliver improved outcomes. However, in many instances, implementation is associated with challenging decision making (47). In addition, much of the evidence of effectiveness is associated with a change in practice and this is undoubtedly true in the case of laboratory medicine, and a most challenging example is point-of-care testing (51). Therefore, in order to deliver the benefits, any decision to change a testing strategy has to be accompanied by a change management strategy that encompasses consultation and reeducation, appropriate reconfiguration of services and resources, and then audit to ensure completion and compliance.

Exercise 8: Identify the changes in clinical practice that might be required to generate the benefits (clinical and economic) from the use of the tests identified in Exercise 1 for a specific clinical setting.

SUMMARY

Good quality evidence enshrined within the principles of evidence-based medicine is the foundation of high-quality clinical care. This is applicable to the maintenance and advancement of laboratory medicine and should be used as the platform for all policy and management decision making. The evidence can be used to inform the breadth and mode of delivery of the service, to establish guidelines, and to audit performance. In addition, it can play a valuable role in identifying the value of the diagnostic service and thereby influence reimbursement strategies to provide the best value for money for the patient and for society.

REFERENCES

1. Sackett DL, Straus SE, Richardson WS, Rosenberg W, Haynes RB, eds. Evidence-based medicine: how to practice and teach EBM. 2nd ed. Edinburgh: Churchill Livingstone, 2000:1–261.
2. Horwitz RI. The dark side of evidence-based medicine. Clev Clin J Med 1996;63:320–3.
3. Charlton BG, Miles A. The rise and fall of EBM. Q J Med 1998;12:371–4.
4. Knottnerus JA, ed. The evidence base of clinical diagnosis. London: BMJ Publishing Group, 2002:1–226.

5. Wyatt JC. Clinical knowledge and practice in the information age. London: Royal Society of Medicine Press, 2001:1–93.

6. Guyatt G, Haynes B, Jaeschke R, Cook D, Greenhalgh T, Meade M, et al. Introduction: the philosophy of evidence-based medicine. In: Guyatt G, Rennie D, eds. User's guide to the medical literature. A manual for evidence-based clinical practice. Chicago: J Am Med Assoc and Archive Journals, American Medical Association, 2002:3–12.

7. Price CP. Evidence-based laboratory medicine. Ned Tijdschr Klin Chem 2001;26:236–42.

8. Sloan FA, ed. Valuing health care: costs, benefits, and effectiveness of pharmaceuticals and other medical technologies. Cambridge: Cambridge University Press, 1995:1–273.

9. Choi BC. Future challenges for diagnostic research: striking a balance between simplicity and complexity. J Epidemiol Community Health 2002;56:334–5.

10. Moons KG, Grobbee DE. Diagnostic studies as multivariable, prediction research. J Epidemiol Community Health 2002;56:337–8.

11. Kilpatrick ES, Holding S. Use of computer terminals on wards to access emergency test results; a retrospective audit. Br Med J 2001;322:1101–3.

12. Bossuyt PMM, Lijmer JG, Mol BWJ. Randomised comparisons of medical tests: sometimes invalid, not always efficient. Lancet 2000;356:1844–7.

13. Feinstein AR. Misguided efforts and future challenges for research on 'diagnostic tests'. J Epidemiol Community Health 2002;56:330–2.

14. Sackett DL, Haynes RB, Guyatt GH, Tugwell P. Clinical epidemiology; a basic science for clinical medicine, 2nd ed. Toronto: Little, Brown, 1991:1–441.

15. Smith R. What clinical information do doctors need? Br Med J 1996;313:1062–8.

16. Reid CK, Lachs MS, Feinstein AR. Use of methodological standards in diagnostic test research. Getting better but still not good. J Am Med Assoc 1995;274:645–51.

17. Lijmer JG, Mol BW, Heisterkamp S, Bonsel GJ, Prins MH, van der Meulen JH, et al. Empirical evidence of design-related bias in studies of diagnostic tests. J Am Med Assoc 1999: 282:1061–6.

18. Mower WR. Evaluating bias and variability in diagnostic test reports. Ann Emerg Med 1999;33:85–91.

19. Hobbs FDR, Delaney BC, Fitzmaurice DA, Wilson S, Hyde CJ, Thorpe GH, et al. A review of near patient testing in primary care. Health Technol Assess 1997;1:1–230.

20. Balk EM, Ioannidis JP, Salem D, Chew PW, Lau J. Accuracy of biomarkers to diagnose acute cardiac ischemia in the emergency department: a meta-analysis. Ann Emerg Med 2001;37:478–94.

21. Munro J, Booth A, Nicholl J. Routine preoperative testing: a systematic review of the evidence. Health Technol Assess 1997;1(12):1–63.

22. Greenhalgh T. Assessing methodological quality. In: How to read a paper: the basics of evidence based medicine, 2nd ed. London: BMJ Publishing Group, 2001:59–75.

23. Sackett DL, Haines RB, The architecture of diagnostic research. Br Med J 2002;321:539–41.

24. Fryback FG, Thornbury JR. The efficacy of diagnostic imaging. Med Decis Making 1991;11:88–94.

25. Price CP. Evidence-based laboratory medicine: supporting decision-making. Clin Chem 2000;46:1041–50.
26. Mackenzie R, Dixon AK. Measuring the effects of imaging: an evaluative framework. Clin Radiol 1995;50:513–8.
27. Van Walraven C, Naylor D. Do we know what inappropriate laboratory utilization is? A systematic review of laboratory clinical audits. J Am Med Assoc 1998;280:550–8.
28. Wong ET. Improving laboratory testing; can we get physicians to focus on outcome? Clin Chem 1995;41:1241–7.
29. Lundberg GD. The need for an outcomes research agenda for clinical laboratory testing. J Am Med Assoc 1998;280:565–6.
30. Antman EM, Lau J, Kupelnick B, Mosteller F, Chalmers TC. A comparison of results of meta-analyses of randomized control trials and recommendations of clinical experts. J Am Med Assoc 1992;268:240–8.
31. Nichols JH, Kickler TS, Dyer K, Humbertson SK, Cooper PC, Maughan WL, et al. Clinical outcomes of point-of-care testing in the intervention radiology and invasive cardiology setting. Clin Chem 2000;46:543–50.
32. Woolf SH, Grol R, Hutchinson A, Eccles M, Grimshaw J. Clinical guidelines: potential benefits, limitations, and harms of clinical guidelines. Br Med J 1999;318:527–30.
33. Sacks DB, Bruns DE, Goldstein DE, Maclaren NK, McDonald JM, Parrott M. Guidelines and recommendations for laboratory analysis in the diagnosis and management of diabetes mellitus. Clin Chem 2002;48:436–72.
34. Lugon M, Secker-Walker J, eds. Clinical governance: making it happen. London: Royal Society of Medicine Press, 1999:1–222.
35. Krumholz H, Herrin J. Quality improvement studies: the need is there but so are the challenges. Am J Med 2000;109:501–3.
36. Davis DA, Thomson MA, Oxman AD, Haynes RB. Changing physician performance: A systematic review of the effect of continuing medical education. J Am Med Assoc 1995;274:700–5.
37. Roe MT, Ohman EM, Pollack CV, Peterson ED, Brandis RG, Harrington RA, et al. Changing the model of care for patients with acute coronary syndromes. Am Heart J (in press).
38. McGovern DPB. Audit. In: McGovern DPB, Valori RM, Summerskill WSM, Levi M, eds. Key topics in evidence-based medicine. Oxford: Bios, 2001:133–6.
39. Inamdar N, Kaplan RS, Bower M. Applying the balanced scorecard in healthcare provider organizations. J Healthc Manag 2002;47:179–95.
40. Galloway M, Nadin L. Benchmarking and the laboratory. J Clin Pathol 2001;54:590–7.
41. Zarbo RJ, Jones BA, Friedberg RC, Valenstein PN, Renner SW, Schitman RB, et al. Q-tracks: a College of American Pathologists program of continuous laboratory monitoring and longitudinal tracking. Arch Pathol Lab Med 2002;126:1036–44.
42. Chang LC, Northcott DN. The NHS performance assessment framework: a 'balanced scorecard' approach? J Manag Med 2002;16:345–58.
43. www.nrmi.org/nrmi_background.html
44. www.renalreg.com
45. www.diabetes.fi/english/programme/programme/chapter14.htm

46. Mushlin AI, Ruchlin HS, Callahan MA. Cost effectiveness of diagnostic tests. Lancet 2001;358:1353–5.
47. Muir Gray JA. Evidence-based healthcare: how to make health policy and management decisions. Edinburgh: Churchill Livingstone, 1997:1–270.
48. O'Brien B, Drummond M, Scott Richardson W, Levine M, Heyland D, Guyatt G. Moving from evidence to action: economic analysis. In: Guyatt G, Rennie D, eds. Users' guides to the medical literature, a manual for evidence-based practice. Chicago: J Am Med Assoc and Archives Journals, American Medical Association, 2002:621–44.
49. Udvarhelyi IS, Rai GA, Epstein AM. Cost-effectiveness and cost-benefit analysis in the medical literature: are methods being used correctly? Ann Intern Med 1992;116:238–44.
50. Langer O, Rodriguez DA, Xenakis EM, McFarland MB, Berkus MD, Arrendondo F, et al. Intensified versus conventional management of gestational diabetes. Am J Obstet Gynecol 1994;170:1036–47.
51. Price CP. Point of care testing: potential for tracking disease management outcomes. Dis Manage Health Outcomes 2002;10:749–61.
52. Diabetes Control and Complications Trial Research Group. Lifetime benefits and costs of intensive therapy as practiced in the Diabetes Control and Complications Trial. J Am Med Assoc 1996;276:1409–15.
53. Gray A, Raikou M, McGuire A, Fenn P, Stevens R, Cull C, et al. Cost effectiveness of an intensive blood glucose control policy in patients with type 2 diabetes: economic analysis alongside randomised controlled trail (UKPDS 41). Br Med J 2000;320:1373–8.
54. Wagner EH, Sandhu N, Newton KM, McCulloch DK, Ramsey SD, Grothaus LC. Effect of improved glycemic control on health care costs and utilization. J Am Med Assoc 2001;285:182–9.
55. Zarich S, Bradley K, Seymour J, Ghali W, Traboulsi A, Mayall ID, et al. Impact of troponin T determinations of hospital resource utilization and costs in the evaluation of patients with suspected myocardial ischemia. Am J Cardiol 2001;88:732–6.
56. Giles W, Bisits A, Know M, Madsen G, Smith R. The effect of fetal fibronectin testing on admissions to a tertiary maternal-fetal medicine unit and cost savings. Am J Obstet Gynecol 2000;182:439–42.
57. Howell MR, Quinn TC, Brathwaite W, Gaydos CA. Screening women for chlamydia trachomatis in family planning clinics. Sex Trans Dis 1998;25:108–17.

Index